Praise for **Jorge Cruise**

"I'm eternally grateful to Jorge for creating a simple lifestyle plan."

— **Christiane Northrup, M.D.,**
#1 *New York Times* best-selling author of *The Wisdom of Menopause*

*"Eat well without dieting or going to the gym with
Jorge's strategies for breakfast, lunch, and dinner."*

— **Mehmet Oz, M.D.,**
host of *The Dr. Oz Show*

*"Jorge Cruise gets it right by eliminating excessive sugar and processed carbohydrates.
His recipes make eating smart easy. I recommend them highly."*

— **Andrew Weil, M.D.,**
Director of the Arizona Center for Integrative Medicine,
University of Arizona, and author of *Why Our Health Matters*

*"Jorge knows, as do I, that excess sugar in our diets is among
the most important factors conspiring against our waistlines and our health."*

— **David Katz, M.D.,**
director and co-founder of Yale University's Prevention Research Center
and nutrition columnist for *O, The Oprah Magazine*

*"The message is simple: eating fat does not make you fat; rather,
eating the right types of fat can help you lose fat. Make a few simple changes
to your lifestyle and start losing your belly fat today."*

— **Terry Grossman, M.D.,**
co-author of *Transcend: Nine Steps to Living Well Forever*

The
AGING
CURE™

Other Books by JORGE CRUISE

The Belly Fat Cure™

The Belly Fat Cure™ *Diet*

The Belly Fat Cure™ *Sugar & Carb Counter*

The Belly Fat Cure™ *Fast Track*

The Belly Fat Cure™ *Quick Meals*

Body at Home™

The 12-Second Sequence™

The 3-Hour Diet™

The 3-Hour Diet™ *Cookbook*

The 3-Hour Diet™ *for Teens*

The 3-Hour Diet™ *On-the-Go*

8 Minutes in the Morning®

8 Minutes in the Morning®: *Extra-Easy Weight Loss*

8 Minutes in the Morning®: *Flat Belly*

8 Minutes in the Morning®: *Lean Hips and Thin Thighs*

Please visit:

Hay House USA: **www.hayhouse.com**®
Hay House Australia: **www.hayhouse.com.au**
Hay House UK: **www.hayhouse.co.uk**
Hay House South Africa: **www.hayhouse.co.za**
Hay House India: **www.hayhouse.co.in**

The AGING CURE™

Reverse 10 years in one week with the FAT-MELTING CARB SWAP™

JORGE CRUISE

HAY HOUSE, INC.
Carlsbad, California • New York City
London • Sydney • Johannesburg
Vancouver • Hong Kong • New Delhi

Published and distributed in the United States by: Hay House, Inc.: www.hayhouse.com • **Published and distributed in Australia by:** Hay House Australia Pty. Ltd.: www.hayhouse.com.au • **Published and distributed in the United Kingdom by:** Hay House UK, Ltd.: www.hayhouse.co.uk • **Published and distributed in the Republic of South Africa by:** Hay House SA (Pty), Ltd.: www.hayhouse.co.za • **Distributed in Canada by:** Raincoast: www.raincoast.com • **Published in India by:** Hay House Publishers India: www.hayhouse.co.in

All photos and illustrations courtesy of JorgeCruise.com, Inc.

<u>The JorgeCruise.com, Inc., team:</u> *Creative editor and executive assistant:* **Michelle McGowen/JorgeCruise.com, Inc.** • *Managing director:* **Oliver Stephenson/JorgeCruise.com, Inc.** • *Legal:* **Kristin Young Rayder/JorgeCruise.com, Inc.** • *Creative Writers:* **Evan Dollard** and **Blair Atkins/JorgeCruise.com, Inc.** • *Personal assistant:* **Kristin Penne/JorgeCruise.com, Inc.**

TRADEMARKS

The Belly Fat Cure	3-Hour Diet	Controlled Tension
The BellyFatCure.com	3HourDiet.com	Jorge Cruise
Carb Swap System	8 Minutes in the Morning	JorgeCruise.com
S/C Value	Super Carbs	Time-Based Nutrition
Body at Home	Fat-Melting Carb Swap	Tasty Carb Swaps
Ulitmate Carb Swap	Be in Control	Restorative Proteins
Everyday Carb Swap	12-Second Sequence	The Aging Cure
12Second.com		

Library of Congress Control Number: 2012946453

ISBN: 978-1-4019-3715-7
Digital ISBN: 978-1-4019-3716-4

16 15 14 13   4 3 2 1
1st edition, January 2013

Printed in China

To Dr. Mehmet Oz,
for showing me that hidden sugar truly is
the #1 way we shorten our "warranty."

Contents

Welcome xi

1 **Cure Aging in One Week!** 1

2 **The FAT-MELTING CARB SWAP™** 11

3 **The One-Week Challenge and Beyond** 27

4 **FAT-MELTING CARB SWAP™ Recipes** 47

5 **FAT-MELTING CARB SWAP™ Products** . . . 159

6 **Fat-Melting Exercises** 223

7 **Frequently Asked Questions (FAQs)** 229

Index of Meals 240
Bibliography 241
Acknowledgments 249
About the Author 250

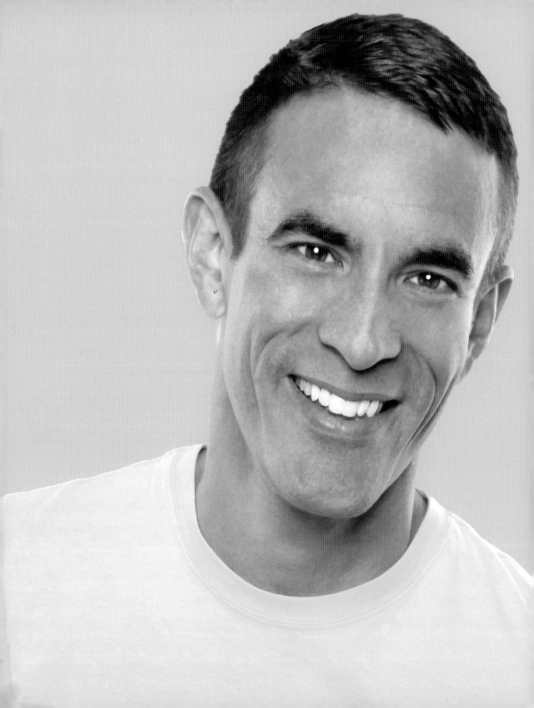

Dear Friend,

For years, experts have told you that you cannot avoid the signs of aging, and if you want to look and feel younger, you must resort to surgeries, creams, or expensive vitamins. Others have told you to simply give up and face the reality of your aging. They were **WRONG!** I am thrilled to share the truth with you. **The one critical solution, the true key to anti-aging, is a diet that avoids hidden sugar and is rich in antioxidants.**

Excessive weight is the number one reason why our bodies look old and feel sluggish. The good news is that there is a solution. You can look and feel vibrant by making a few simple lifestyle changes. The only true anti-aging secret is to protect yourself from the inside out by keeping insulin levels low and antioxidant levels high.

Many popular, supposedly healthy antioxidant-rich sources are loaded with hidden sugar and actually accelerate aging. With this book, you will automatically avoid hidden sugar and uncover the proven power of antioxidants to instantly reverse the effects of aging, increase your life span, and cure belly fat—guaranteed.

What's the secret? I call it the FAT-MELTING CARB SWAP™, and it is the most powerful tool for your ultimate success that I have ever shared. I've made reversing 10 years in one week effortless. Since my 40th birthday, I have been following this all-new method, and it works like magic! I now look and feel younger and have all-day energy. I've never felt better.

I look forward to helping you out on this fresh start to your life as you discover the true cure to aging.

Your coach,

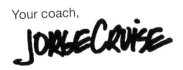

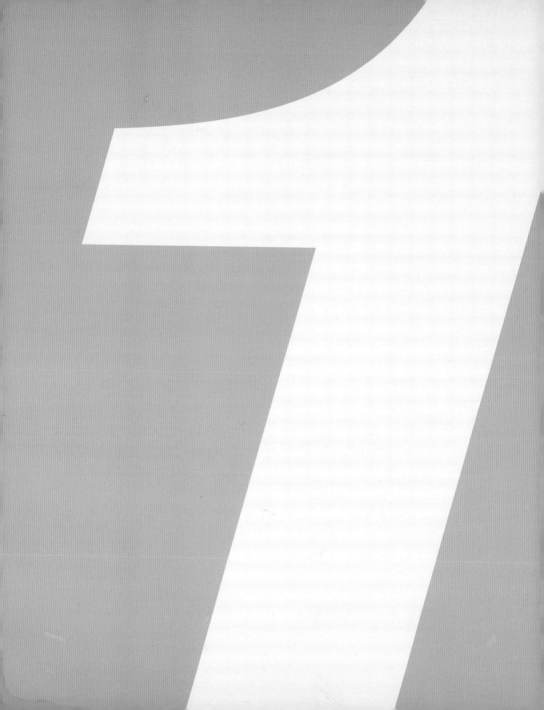

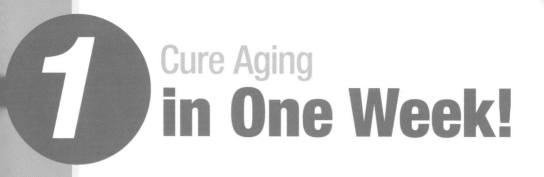

1 Cure Aging
in One Week!

*"I am a single mother of three, and I lost 85 pounds—
I look younger and feel better than ever before.
If I can do it, anyone can!"*

—ADRIENNE DeMOND, LOST 85 LBS.

For the next few pages I want you to forget everything you've been taught about aging, life expectancy, and your waistline. Now imagine looking up to 10 years younger in one week and keeping a smaller waist for the rest of your very long life. What would that freedom mean to you?

Believe it or not, that is the future ahead of you. You will not find the cure to aging in a lotion, at the end of a Botox needle, or in expensive surgeries. The true key to aging more slowly begins in your kitchen. Give me a week in your kitchen, and I will show you how to look younger, feel younger, and lose up to 9 lbs. of belly fat with the most delicious food you've ever eaten! I want to empower you to live well forever. This book will show you how.

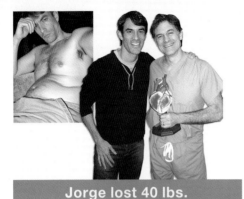

Age: 40
Height: 6'0"
Belly Inches Lost: 5"

Growing up, my best friend was food. I looked forward to hearing the ice-cream truck each day, and at night, I constantly begged my parents for second helpings of desserts. By the time I was a teen, my appendix burst and I almost died. It wasn't until I met Dr. Mehmet Oz that I was awakened to the fact that too much sugar was the heart of the problem and a significant contributor to aging.

My quest became satisfying my sweet tooth without all the hidden sugar. Because of this I was able to create the CARB SWAP™. I realized I didn't have to eat less or give up all the foods I loved—thank goodness!—in order to lose weight and stay young. Since then, it has become my passion to educate people on how they can lose weight and still eat the tasty foods they enjoy.

BEST TIP FOR SUCCESS:
Never feel like you have to give up your sweet tooth. With my CARB SWAP™, you will always be able to find an option to keep you satisfied without eating less or feeling like you're dieting.

In a recent article published by *USA Today,* industry analysts projected that anti-aging will become a $115 billion industry by 2015. That's "billion" with a "b" . . . and that number represents the U.S. market exclusively. As a culture we've put a premium on looking younger longer. Our nation is completely obsessed, and I'll be honest: I'm not immune!

I turned 40 this year, and you'd think it was a mild tragedy. I found myself spending more time in front of the mirror meticulously evaluating my appearance. I felt like Detective Jorge Cruise on the case to uncover all evidence acquit me of my age. I measured my waistline, took the magnifying glass my face for skin clarity and wrinkles, and then interviewed possible accomplices. A few of my close friends were lining for cosmetic enhancements, skin peels and hormone treatments. A handful other well-intentioned friends sided the theory of "aging gracefully" and grin-and-bear-it technique.

"Age is just a number," I kept hearing. It made me cringe.

In truth, I didn't want to be "old news." My whole career has been about helping women and men effortlessly achieve optimal health by getting rid of their belly fat. I don't believe looks are everything, but I know that people pay attention to appearance. The last thing I wanted was to get cast aside for someone who looked younger. My age was causing me a bit of panic. I had a growing fear of rejection.

If you're like me, you've experienced a similar "crisis of aging." Are we crazy? Should we simply put our desire to look and feel younger on the shelf and "let the process happen"? Is it time to ignore the extra inches on our waistline rather than finally drop the belly fat once and for all? The answer to all those questions is no, and I'll tell you exactly why.

The desire to look our best is biological. Humans equate beauty with true health. I discovered that waist circumference is not only the first gauge of someone's attractiveness, it has also been a measurement of true health since the dawn of the human race. A woman could evaluate a man's testosterone levels based on his waist size and determine whether or not he was a viable mate. Added inches on a man's waistline convert testosterone to estrogen, resulting in a lower sperm count. Similarly,

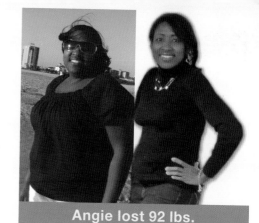

Angie lost 92 lbs.

Age: 40
Height: 5'3"
Belly Inches Lost: 10"

I didn't intend to lose weight. Instead, I came across *The Aging Cure*™ when I was looking for a cookbook and the recipes looked great. I began cooking from it and realized that I was losing weight. I figured it was temporary, but I was wrong. With the pounds went all my bad eating and drinking habits. I applied what I learned and found a new me.

I am a 40-year-old woman and have more energy than I did at 14! Simple tasks such as putting my shoes on, walking, and sleeping used to be a struggle for me. Now I can walk for miles without tiring and sleep in any position with comfort. Shopping for clothes used to make me depressed, but I can now slide clothes onto my body without any hassle. It feels great to be able to choose an outfit off the rack and have it fit the first time I try it on.

I don't think it was easy for my children to live with an overweight mother, and I longed for them to see me at a smaller size. I am so grateful that I came across Jorge's book that day. Now I see pride in my kids' eyes when they look at me.

BEST TIP FOR SUCCESS:
Don't be afraid to think outside of the book! I've come up with so many tasty meals myself that I've made over and over again.

mate. Added inches on a man's waistline convert testosterone to estrogen, resulting in a lower sperm count. Similarly, men identified excess belly fat on a woman as an indicator of either pregnancy or hormonal imbalance. We are hardwired to associate external beauty with internal health.

Obviously, you don't need to be living in a cave or to be in the business of finding a mate to understand the principle here: our biological instinct is to determine health and beauty based on physical indicators. If you think you're crazy for wanting to look and feel young, let me assure you that you're absolutely normal.

Additionally, many of the supposed "signs of aging" are actually the result of poor dietary health. The truth is there are two primary dietary components that will make you look older faster. The first component ages you more quickly because you're getting too much of it, and the second ages you more quickly because you're not getting enough of it.

As it turns out, the same supervillain responsible for extra inches on your waistline is also leading the assault against your appearance: hidden sugar. Time and time again I hear a new client say, "I avoid sugar," "I enjoy my coffee without a packet of sweetener," or "When I was a kid I ate lots of sugary foods, but I've stopped eating candy bars and ice cream now." This is why I call it "hidden"—to help you realize that this sneaky little devil is not just in packets of added sugar, ice cream, or candy bars, but often in the common foods and products that you would least expect.

The second dietary component is something you need *more* of: antioxidants. These microscopic miracle workers are found predominantly in veggies, herbs, and spices and they help fight against dangerous free radicals and age-accelerating oxidation.

I've been privileged throughout my career as a fitness expert to connect with a handful of trusted experts who have been kind enough over the years to share their insights with me. I like to refer to them as my "Inner Circle": Dr. Mehmet Oz, Dr. Christiane Northrup, and Dr. Nicholas Perricone. These contemporary wizards of true health and beauty agree that aging more slowly begins in the kitchen, and that consuming whole foods high in antioxidants is key to overall health.

My good friend Dr. Oz, who is always an inspiration to me, says that antioxidants are not only beneficial to our diet, but also essential for health. He notes that antioxidants protect your skin from hazardous free-radical damage by promoting healthy development of collagen and elastin. These proteins make up your skin, and they must be kept healthy to help it remain smooth, flexible, and wrinkle-free. This is why antioxidants are crucial for decreasing the appearance of wrinkles.

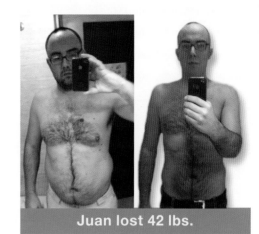

Juan lost 42 lbs.

Age: 40
Height: 6'1"
Belly Inches Lost: 8.5"

For over 15 years I didn't pay much attention to the food I was eating. Whenever I felt hungry, I snacked on junk food without thinking about it. But thanks to Jorge, I have totally changed my eating habits. Before *The Aging Cure*™, I felt heavy and tired, and I even had difficulty breathing when I lay in bed. Now I can play basketball for an hour without feeling tired! I have energy all day long.

BEST TIP FOR SUCCESS:
Keep it simple. You can find vegetables, cheese, and eggs wherever you live. Everything you need to shed the weight is right in your neighborhood grocery store. I live in Spain, and I can still make this program work without using any of the specialty products Jorge recommends in his books.

Similarly, Dr. Perricone is emphatic that what you eat is key to how young yo[u] look. His research has revealed that high-sugar diets result in *advanced glycatio[n] end products* (AGEs) that are linked not only to visible signs of aging, but to diseas[e] as well. He goes so far to say that "Fighting AGEs and the related inflammation i[s] the best strategy we have to combat disease." I explain more of this in Chapter 2.

My dear friend Dr. Northrup also praises antioxidants for their ability to balanc[e] hormones, which is important during menopause. She emphasizes their importanc[e] in protecting your body through combating cellular damage from free radical[s] which is a known contributor to conditions such as heart disease and cance[r.] Dr. Northrup observes that additional benefits of antioxidants include the reductio[n] of visible signs of aging, radiant skin, protection from sun damage, and preventio[n] of varicose veins.

The truth is that you can have incredible years of life ahead of you in whic[h] you look and feel your very best. I believe you can be healthy and active into yo[ur] 80s, 90s, and even 100s! If you find yourself starting to think that the extra pound[s,] deeper wrinkles, and seemingly endless fatigue are natural pieces of the aging pu[z-]zle, then I'm here to guide you to the truth.

It wasn't until I uncovered the science of *The Belly Fat Cure*™ that I was fina[lly] able to overcome my continual struggle to keep off belly fat long term. I also lo[ok] and feel younger now, and I want the same for you. I've come face-to-face with hu[n-]dreds of clients over the years who nearly gave up on experiencing true health a[nd] a smaller waist. I know what it's like to be 40 lbs. overweight and feel unattracti[ve.] I always seemed to have low energy and achy joints; worst of all, my self-este[em] was at an all-time low. It was then that this thought crossed my mind: *Maybe this [is] simply my body getting older.* That was before my grandmother passed away, at t[he] age of 102. Just try to have a conversation about the woes of aging with a centen[ar-]ian; you will never get a word in edgewise!

If you're like many of my clients, there's just one roadblock that is stopping you fro[m] transforming your appearance and waistline: a seemingly uncontrollable attitude of defe[at]

To be truly successful, it is essential that you *believe* you can succeed. I want to help you trade in all negativity for a positive attitude.

The Vicious Cycle Threatening Your Youth

A recent study revealed that more than half of working adults are overstressed. Of course, I don't need a study to prove that—I can take a quick glance at my own life and become convinced! I'm all too familiar with the relationship between stress and nutrition.

Researchers at the American Psychological Association confirmed that everyday emotional stressors such as work and family can lead to impulsive eating choices. The remorse from such choices then adds emotional stress that leads to more impulsive eating. You can see how this vicious cycle could rapidly increase your visible age and waistline, and put your life span in jeopardy, especially when the foods you're reaching for are loaded with hidden sugar and low in antioxidants.

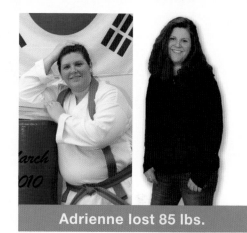

Adrienne lost 85 lbs.

Age: 33
Height: 5'4"
Belly Inches Lost: 15"

Although I had been pretty active, I had also been "chunky" all my life. At age 30, I couldn't walk up a flight of stairs without nearly collapsing. I began Tae Kwon Do, which helped me lose some weight, but after getting divorced, I found myself far bigger. *The Aging Cure*™ showed me that simple changes—such as drinking Zevia instead of Pepsi—could help me shed major pounds.

I am a single mother of three, and I'm so thankful for the way that Jorge's plan has transformed not just my own life, but the lives of my kids. They have become aware of serving sizes and sugar grams at a young age and excitedly point out how they can hug me "all the way around" now! Thanks, Jorge, for assisting my family and me in living a healthier life.

BEST TIP FOR SUCCESS:
Get your children involved with your weight-loss journey as well. They will learn valuable lessons they can use later on in life to prevent them from packing on the pounds!

It's true that there are many circumstances over which you have little to no control that can trigger emotional stress. In order to reach the point of personal strength and empowerment to respond in healthy ways to these stressors, I recommend focusing on what you *can* control. That begins with my FAT-MELTING CARB SWAP™. Studies show that less belly fat makes you feel more attractive. That's not vanity, it's science, and I believe it's incredibly important. Empowerment allows you to live authentically and, therefore, up to your fullest potential. Truly, the more inner confidence you achieve, the greater impact you'll have in your relationships.

I know what it's like to lean on carbs for comfort when caught in that cycle of stress eating, remorse, and weight gain. When you're in the thick of it, every day is a struggle. I can honestly say that dropping the belly fat allowed me to struggle significantly less than I ever had before in my life. Once I experienced the confidence boost that comes with a smaller waist, I began to recognize that my insecurities were largely rooted in an inability to live authentically from the inside out. I've also learned to surround myself with trusted friends for accountability.

There is a quote from civil-rights leader Howard Thurman that always keeps me motivated: "Don't ask yourself what the world needs. Ask yourself what makes you come alive and then go do that. Because what the world needs is people who have come alive."

As a coach, I believe the answer to the question "What makes you come alive?" begins with the empowerment of a healthy appearance and enough energy to make it through each day. Many of my clients have faced the social stigma that comes with extra weight. For some, simply leaving the house to go for a walk causes them to feel a sense of embarrassment. For others, adversity is present in the home. I've heard a number of stories that truly break my heart: roller-coaster dieting while enduring the stress of being a working mother or having a perpetually unsupportive spouse. Whatever the case may be, I know it's a very real struggle. I also know with absolute certainty that it's not your fault.

I can't remove the adversity surrounding you. I can, however, help you rewrite your success story starting today. Your path leads you to younger-looking skin, a healthier body, and a smaller waist. My magical FAT-MELTING CARB SWAP™ will empower you to become the best, most confident version of yourself.

The kitchen is your true anti-aging center. In the next chapter I will unveil for the first time the most powerful CARB SWAP™ I've ever created. It will bring instant balance to your fat-controlling hormone, insulin; help reverse glycation, which causes the formation of fine lines and wrinkles; and provide you all the positive health and beauty benefits of antioxidants. You can look and feel younger this week, and effortlessly drop 10 years in one week with the amazingly powerful FAT-MELTING CARB SWAP™.

It's time to take control of the way you look and feel. If you're ready to transform your life for a fresh start, keep reading!

2

The Fat-Melting
Carb Swap™

"*I worked out for years and even ran several marathons, but it wasn't until I started following The Aging Cure™ that I achieved the bikini body I had always dreamed of. These days, when I shop with my two teenage daughters, we all wear the same size!*"

—AMY VAN ARKEL, LOST 37 LBS.

Now that you've set aside all doubt, it's time for me to unveil the revolutionary tool that will reduce the visible signs of aging while you effortlessly drop inches from your waist—the FAT-MELTING CARB SWAP™. I consider it the hero of anti-aging, and I'm thrilled to share with you the cutting-edge science that will show you how to become the best version of yourself. I believe that the story of your health, vitality, and waistline is about to get very exciting.

Of course—as in any great tale—every hero has a villain. Whenever I watch a new movie, I love that turning point when, against all odds, the bad guy finally gets what he deserves and the hero lives happily ever after.

As a fitness expert who has helped millions reach their goal weight for over a decade, I can promise you one thing with absolute certainty: Your age, health, and waistline all have the same villain. His name is "hidden sugar." As opposed to the movies, in real life the stakes are a lot higher . . . cue the suspenseful music.

The Villain in Your Home

The villain I'm talking about here is not in some faraway place secretly plotting against your skin and waistline. He's actually staked out very close to you. In fact, if you're like the majority of my clients, then it's likely he's already infiltrated your home.

The average American consumes around 130 grams or more of sugar daily! Take a stroll into your kitchen and explore the contents of your fridge and pantry, and then read the nutrition labels on some of the common food items you consume each week. How many grams of sugar are in that key-lime yogurt? What about your morning cereal? And that carton of orange juice and gallon of milk? It's likely that one serving of each of those items exceeds the number of sugar grams you should be consuming for the entire day.

In truth, sugar is everywhere . . . and often in the products that you'd least expect. That's why I call it "hidden." It's not as though you're reaching for a jar of cookies or pint of ice cream, or sprinkling your meals with packets of sugar. Those are sources of sugar of which you're well aware. But it hides out in many of the foods you believe to be healthy and FYI, it's almost always in those that are labeled "low fat" or "low calorie."

In an interview I conducted with Dr. Perricone, he contended that the rise of glucose levels due to an excess consumption of sugar—including that found in everyday "healthy" items such as skim milk and yogurt—can result in high blood-sugar levels that can last three to four days. The effects impact not only how old you look on the outside (through wrinkles, sagging skin, etc.), but also your physical health and organ function. It is like increasing your age both externally and internally.

The Impact of Hidden Sugar

Traditionally, every bad guy has a lair. It's his place to hide out and come up with kinds of terrible plans to try to ruin things for the world. In the narrative of your waistline this bad guy doesn't have one lair, but hundreds of thousands. In order to fully grasp the dastardly character in the plot against your age and belly, let me first set the stage.

Excess sugar consumption is responsible for elevated levels of the fat-controlling hormone insulin. When you consume sugar, it triggers a release of insulin that locks in belly fat so you can't lose those extra inches. Those inches are incredibly hazardous to your health.

Excess sugar consumption also triggers two harmful conditions in your body that are responsible for accelerating the signs of aging and adding inches to your waistline. The first is a process known as *glycation.* Glycation occurs when a sugar molecule binds to a protein molecule, which creates "advanced glycation end products," also known as AGEs. When glycation causes collagen and elastin (proteins responsible for healthy skin) to cross-link and create AGEs, it results in stiff, inflexible skin and the formation of fine lines and wrinkles. An abundance of AGEs in your body will accelerate the signs of aging and wreak havoc on your looks as well as your overall health.

The second condition, which is aggravated by glycation, is free-radical damage. The glycation process produces a continuous stream of free radicals, which are unstable molecules that bond to other molecules in your tissues, causing damage to cells and their DNA. Then AGEs induce oxidative stress, which is when oxidants overwhelm the body's ability to detoxify with antioxidants. Free radicals also stimulate inflammation throughout the body and can result in cell and tissue damage and even cell death. The outcome of all this damage is not only disease, such as autoimmune disorders and cancer, but discolored skin, wrinkles, and just a general lack of radiance. As Dr. Perricone observes, "Sugar can rob you of your youth, health, and beauty." It is imperative to minimize the number of free radicals in your body if you want to slow down the aging process and attain optimal health.

WEIGHING IN ON ORAC

Oxygen Radical Absorbance Capacity, or ORAC, is the standard by which antioxidant values are measured in food. There are several types of antioxidants, which can be found predominantly in fruits, vegetables, spices, and herbs. While ORAC is certainly a great starting point, it does have limitations. For starters, ORAC measures antioxidant properties collectively rather than individually.

Consider spinach for a moment. The ORAC value of raw spinach is estimated to be around 1515 for a single ounce. Spinach is known to be an excellent source of several antioxidants, including vitamin C; however, it does not weigh the value of that antioxidant specifically against all others. Another food rich in vitamin C is strawberries, which has an ORAC value of 4302 per ounce. At first glance, you might think, *Well, why don't I just eat loads of strawberries every day instead of spinach?* Honestly, it's a fair question, and I get it. Have you ever been spinach picking? Neither have I! On the other hand, I have been strawberry picking, and if I'm completely honest I would much rather devour a basket of those sweet, juicy, ruby-red delicacies rather than munch on a plate of raw spinach.

Unfortunately, there are a couple things that ORAC can't predict. The first you might have guessed already: like all fruit, strawberries are concentrated sources of fructose that, despite being a "natural" source of sugar, triggers a release of insulin that locks in belly fat. This visceral fat causes chronic inflammation that puts you at risk for disease. ORAC does not measure the benefit of free-radical absorption against the potential harm of elevated insulin as it relates to glycation and belly fat.

Second, the source of the antioxidant appears to be a factor in overall effectiveness. A study conducted at the Jean Mayer USDA Human Nutrition Research Center on Aging measured the effect of antioxidant-rich diets on cognitive function and health in rats. Each furry group was given a diet similar in antioxidant properties, but varying in source. The control group was given a plain diet. Of the remaining rats, one group's food was fortified with spinach extract, the next group received strawberry extract, and the final group had vitamin E. When tested at the rodent equivalent of middle age, the group receiving spinach extract had much better long-term memory and learning ability than any of the others. While it is difficult to know precisely how a particular antioxidant-rich food will react in the human body, what is absolutely considered valuable is to include several sources of antioxidants in as many of your meals as possible.

ORAC is a valuable measurement, but it's definitely not the final say on the most beneficial sources of antioxidants. That's why I consider ORAC a guiding light. It's a great resource to identify antioxidant-rich foods and make informed, *The Aging Cure*™–approved decisions every day.

Your Waistline Predicts Your Life Span

Studies conducted by the *New England Journal of Medicine* correlate one's life span directly to the measurement of one's waistline. Startlingly, a study by Harvard Medical School linked higher waist circumference to premature death in women. That's why the FAT-MELTING CARB SWAP™ addresses not only the visible signs of aging that result from glycation, but also the extra inches around your waist.

The problem is more than skin deep. Lurking beneath the unwanted inches you can see and feel is a more dangerous type of fat wreaking havoc on your health. You see, there are two types of body fat: *subcutaneous* and *visceral*. Many of my clients are most familiar with subcutaneous fat, which is the visible type of fat residing just below the skin, measurable with a simple pinch. If you're like me, this is what you're most concerned about. When I was overweight, my main concern was losing the extra inches I could see and feel. What I didn't realize is that visceral fat is actually more dangerous.

Visceral fat resides deep in your midsection and is invisible to the eye. This dangerous fat surrounds vital organs and causes chronic inflammation. That's when things get scary. Visceral fat triggers immune cells to secrete substances known as *cytokines* that become hazardous to your health over time.

It's important to recognize that cytokines aren't trying to act like bad guys. These substances are proteins, peptides, or glycoproteins secreted by certain cells that carry signals between other cells. Essentially, cytokines act as the immune system's messengers and regulators and are a natural part of the immune system's inflammation response to various types of physiological stress.

The problem is that your body recognizes visceral fat as a "threat" to your body in constant need of repair. Elevated levels of cytokines in the bloodstream have been linked to several health risks. Studies supported by medical experts from both the Mayo Clinic and Harvard University connect belly fat to three of the leading killers out there: heart disease, cancer, and type 2 diabetes. In order to significantly reduce your risk of disease and enjoy

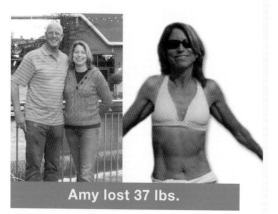

Amy lost 37 lbs.

Age: 43
Height: 5'5"
Belly Inches Lost: 8"

I worked out for years and even ran several marathons, but it wasn't until I started following *The Aging Cure*™ that I achieved the bikini body I had always dreamed of. As much as I exercised, my incorrect food choices kept me from losing weight. When I began my journey, I weighed 155 lbs., and this past summer I was down to 118 lbs. I definitely feel younger, too. These days, when I shop with my two teenage daughters, we swap clothes over the dressing-room doors because we all wear about the same size! I cannot tell you how many people ask me how I lost the weight. I sing the praises of *The Aging Cure*™ to all.

BEST TIP FOR SUCCESS:
Slowly incorporate walking into your day. The fresh air and new atmosphere helps you relax and really enjoy life!

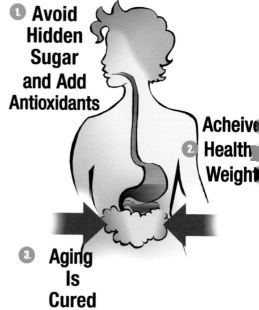

1. **Avoid Hidden Sugar and Add Antioxidants**

Acheive Healthy Weight

2.

3. **Aging Is Cured**

a longer, healthier life, you must lose those extra inches.

The most effective way to reduce visceral fat is to avoid hidden sugar with my FAT-MELTING CARB SWAP™. By doing so, you will significantly lower your risk for those three top killers, and increase your chances for a long and healthy life. Additionally, you'll significantly reduce the continual stress of subcutaneous fat on your skeletal, muscular, and cardiovascular systems, which will decrease your risk of chronic back pain and sore joints.

Antioxidants: Your Knights in Shining Armor

As you now know, sugar in all its forms is responsible for accelerated aging and added inches. That's why, first and foremost, my FAT-MELTING CARB SWAP™ promotes the powerful preventive remedy of avoiding hidden sugar to keep insulin moderated and to protect against harmful oxidation. If avoiding hidden sugar is the defensive measure, then antioxidants are the offensive that keeps you healthy. That's why I consider antioxidants your knights in shining armor.

Antioxidants are so named because of their ability to counter free radicals that infiltrate your bloodstream. Simply put, an antioxidant is a substance such as vitamin C or vitamin B$_1$ (thiamin) that inhibits destructive oxidizing agents in a living organism. Additionally, these microscopic miracle workers enhance circulation and increase white-blood-cell count. And as a bonus, items rich in antioxidants are typically rich in other nutrients.

Each of my FAT-MELTING CARB SWAP™ recipes is designed with both defensive and offensive measures in mind. In truth, if you're regulating your insulin by avoiding hidden sugar, you automatically reduce your risk of oxidation. Still, I've found it is valuable for overall health to ensure that every meal contains a balanced amount of nutrient-rich antioxidant food sources.

However, there's just one tiny problem . . .

If you were to take a trip to your local grocery store to check out the latest lineup of popular antioxidant products and looked at how much sugar was in each one, the numbers would shock you. The first time I took a close look at the nutrition labels on popular antioxidant products (knowing what I do now about the dangers of hidden sugar), I couldn't believe it. The packaging was bright, fun, and—dare I say it—downright sexy, but numbers told a darker story. One curvy little 16-ounce bottle of a popular pomegranate juice, for instance, had 58 grams of hidden sugar.

"Fifty-eight?!"

I nearly dropped the bottle. I wanted to run over to the nearest PA to make an announcement to the entire store: "Clean up on aisle 2!"

I've always wanted to say that. That's definitely how I would've started. Then would've launched into a passionate tirade that went something like this:

"Attention, shoppers . . . you've been duped! That well-lit fridge over by the produc with its colorful collection of antioxidant juices is a marketing myth. Every one of thos bottles is loaded with hidden sugar. These products are contributing to inflammation your body rather than decreasing harmful oxidation in your blood. They are making yo more susceptible to illness rather than reducing your risk for disease. Steer clear! Now w somebody please bring a mop to aisle 2 . . . "

Of course, I decided it would not be best to engage in a wrestling match with the sto manager for a few seconds of grocery-store glory. I had a better idea: put it in this book

The FAT-MELTING CARB SWAP™

My FAT-MELTING CARB SWAP™ is the remedy to accelerated signs of aging a extra inches on the waistline. It brings instant balance to the fat-controlling horme insulin by telling you exactly when and what to eat to avoid hidden sugar, so your be can burn belly fat. This is key to increasing your life span and finally being the healthi most vibrant version of you.

The core of the FAT-MELTING CARB SWAP™ is to avoid hidden sugar with ant dant-rich meals. The principle of swapping one meal option for another is familiar to th who have been following the Belly Fat Cure. To keep things simple, I have put mea two categories: Age Less and Age More. Unlike the traditional CARB SWAPS™ four my original *Belly Fat Cure*™ book, though, swapping one antioxidant food for anoth not as simple as swapping out a pie from Pizza Hut in favor of one of my pita pizza pes. Here's why: high-sugar, antioxidant-rich foods typically do not have an Age Les ternative that will preserve the taste integrity of a meal. For example, I can't swap a N juice with pureed garlic. (Well, I guess I could do that, but it would be kind of gross.

have a hunch that my conversations with friends would start getting cut short!) Since it's
ot a simple "swap this antioxidant for that one," the FAT-MELTING CARB SWAP™ is all
bout creating an entire meal.

Imagine two similar lunches. The first is a tuna sandwich on Milton's multigrain bread
nd a glass of cranberry juice on the side. The second is a tuna sandwich on sprouted grain
read with pepper-jack cheese and fresh baby spinach leaves, with a handful of raspber-
es on the side and an unsweetened iced tea with fresh mint. The first meal will add inches
) your waistline by hiking up your insulin with the heaping servings of hidden sugar in the
read and fruit juice. The second is not only Age Less, since there's very little sugar, but
ou will also be satisfied with great taste; maintain a stable insulin level; and invigorate your
ody with healthy antioxidants found in the fresh spinach, raspberries, and tea.

That is the power of the FAT-MELTING CARB SWAP™ at work. The best part is I've
lready done all the thinking for you. To reduce the physical effects of aging while reach-
g your goal weight fast, simply live by the S/C Value—the Sugar and Carb Value—of
5/6. Here's how it works: Consume up to 15 grams of sugar and up to 6 servings of
arbohydrates a day. As you do, you will easily reduce your belly fat by bringing balance
) your insulin level.

A typical carb serving would be represented by a ¼ cup of brown rice or a slice of
read. Here's how to measure a serving during a meal:

- 0–4 carbohydrate grams = not counted
- 5–20 carbohydrate grams = 1 serving
- 21–40 carbohydrate grams = 2 servings
- 41–60 carbohydrate grams = 3 servings

Each of my FAT-MELTING CARB SWAP™ recipes automatically keeps you on track for
5/6 by ensuring that each serving has an S/C Value of 5/2 or less. You can enjoy three of
nese recipes a day—plus two tasty, 0/0 snacks—and effortlessly drop all the belly fat and
ge more slowly. It's simple and completely delicious! However, first you should commit to
ny One-Week Challenge in the next Chapter. During your One-Week Menu, you don't need

TOP AGE LESS ANTIOXIDANT-RICH FOODS

Nuts and Seeds

almonds (¼ cup): 0/1

flaxseed (¼ cup): 0/1

hazelnuts (¼ cup): 1/1

macadamia nuts (¼ cup): 1/1

pecans (¼ cup): 1/0

pistachios (¼ cup): 2/1

pumpkin seeds (¼ cup): 0/0

sesame seeds (¼ cup): 0/1

sunflower seeds (¼ cup): 1/1

walnuts (¼ cup): 0/0

Herbs, Spices, and Condiments

basil (5 leaves): 0/0

bay leaf (1 Tbsp.): 0/0

black pepper (1 tsp.): 0/0

capers (1 Tbsp.): 0/0

cayenne pepper (1 tsp.): 0/0

chili powder (1 tsp.): 0/0

cilantro (¼ cup): 0/0

cinnamon (1 tsp.): 0/0

coriander (1 tsp.): 0/0

cumin (1 tsp.): 0/0

curry powder (1 tsp.): 0/0

dill (1 tsp.): 0/0

garlic (1 clove): 0/0

ginger (1 tsp.): 0/0

lemon juice (1 fl. oz.): 1/0

mint (5 leaves): 0/0

nutmeg (1 tsp.): 0/0

oregano (1 tsp.): 0/0

parsley (5 sprigs): 0/0

rosemary (1 tsp.): 0/0

sage (1 tsp.): 0/0

tarragon (1 tsp.): 0/0

thyme (1 tsp.): 0/0

turmeric (1 tsp.): 0/0

Good Fats

avocado (¼ whole): 0/1

coconut, shredded (¼ cup): 1/0

extra-virgin olive oil (1 Tbsp.): 0/0

Vegetables

arugula (1 cup): 0/0

asparagus (3 spears): 1/0

broccoli (½ cup, chopped): 1/0

broccoli sprouts (½ cup): 0/0

brussels sprouts (½ cup): 1/0

cauliflower (½ cup, chopped): 1/0

chives (1 Tbsp., chopped): 0/0

eggplant (½ cup, chopped): 1/0

kale (½ cup, chopped): 0/0

olives (1 oz.): 0/0

onion (¼ cup, chopped): 2/1

romaine lettuce (1 cup, shredded): 1/0

scallions (1 Tbsp., chopped): 0/0

shallots (1 Tbsp., chopped): 1/0

spinach (1 cup): 0/0

turnips (¼ cup): 1/0

Fruit

blueberries (2 Tbsp.): 2/0

strawberries (3 berries): 2/0

Treats

cacao nibs (1 oz.): 0/1

cocoa, unsweetened (1 Tbsp.): 0/0

dark chocolate (1 oz.): 5/1

red wine (5 fl. oz.): 0/0

Beverages

coffee (8 oz.): 0/0

espresso (1 oz): 0/0

green tea (8 oz.): 0/0

o worry about tracking your carbohydrate or sugar servings or calculating your daily S/C alue—all the work has already been done for you! Then, after completing the One-Week Menu, you can easily personalize 15/6 to match your taste and lifestyle. (A great tool to help ou with this is my *Belly Fat Cure*™ *Sugar & Carb Counter,* which contains the S/C Value for housands of items, both those you find in restaurants as well as the grocery store.)

If you're looking to add some antioxidants to your meal, just look to the left. You'll otice that I have included a list of the top Age Less antioxidant-rich foods to help guide ur choices should you decide to track 15/6 on your own after completing my One-Week enu. I recommend including one or more of these items in every meal.

"Makes sense to me, Jorge," you might be saying, "but shouldn't I be counting calories well?"

Great question! I'm thrilled to say the answer is no. Here's why.

top Counting Calories and Age Less

My good friend Gary Taubes—author of *Why We Get Fat and What to Do about It*— ntinues to be a brilliant voice of reason in an industry littered with inaccurate science, Blasters, and cabbage diets. He travels the world to share the cutting-edge research t shows not all calories have the same impact on your body, and why the conventional sdom of "eating less and exercising more" does not work. One of the ways he helps ple understand the complexities of the science begins with this provocative question: you remember the expression, 'work up an appetite'?"

If you were anything like me as a kid, you might have been occasionally asked to "go side and play" while dinner was being made. Not only would that give my mother a come break from my antics, it also ensured I'd be hungry. Turns out that the human y is wired to match energy for energy. Just like playing hide-and-seek before dinner, ninutes of a workout or exercise DVD requires energy. Your body expends calories to you that energy, and the hunger you experience afterward is your body requesting your calorie input match your calorie output.

Consider for a moment *The Biggest Loser* model of weight loss. That program is an extreme application of "calories count." It's no joke on "the ranch," as it's called. Even when the cameras stop rolling, those contestants are on the treadmills with their coaches standing by. Their lives mirror that of a professional athlete in the sense that their full-time job becomes nonstop training for eight hours a day. Unlike professional athletes, however, they're not consuming fuel to optimize their bodies for performance. Instead, contestants are in a perpetual state of energy deficit. When their bodies naturally work up an appetite—as Gary Taubes describes—they suffer through the hunger pains for weeks. I promise you, it is incredibly hard work and absolutely not sustainable. You don't live your life on a fitness ranch. Yes, it makes for great television, but that method is not going to help you personally reach and maintain your goal weight and increase longevity.

The other problem with trying to drop weight with what I call the "calorie myth" is that not all calories are created equal. Food sources from each of the macronutrient categories—carbohydrates, fats, and proteins—all have calories. However, not calories have the same impact on your body. Carbohydrates are the only calories that trigger your pancreas to release insulin.

I call my solution the FAT-MELTING CARB SWAP™ because carbohydrates are the only types of macronutrients that raise the level of insulin, and sugar is a simple carbohydrate. That brings me to another lair of hidden sugar that few of my clients like to talk about: fruit.

Dear Fruit, I Think We Should See Other People . . .

But I still want to be friends! It's a bit of a silly thing to say, I know. Still, I believe that the healthiest relationship you can have with fruit is a sparing one. That's why I consider fruit to be candy . . . nature's candy. While it's true that fruit is a natural, unprocessed source of sweetness, it still contains fructose that raises your blood-sugar levels, just a candy bar does. That's why I always recommend clients eat only one or two servings day of an intact, whole fruit.

"Intact" means a fruit (a handful of berries is ideal!) that has not been processed or juiced. The reason eating whole, intact fruit is critical to successfully curing belly fat is simple: fiber. The "packaging" of a fruit is a healthy source of fiber that acts as a buffer that reduces the impact fructose has on blood-sugar levels. Juicing strips fruit of its fiber, and thus its buffer, allowing fructose to make a beeline for your blood-stream and trigger an insulin spike.

Now you can see the danger of popular antioxidant products. So many of them are just juice (that is, fructose) with minimal fiber. Even though the list of antioxidant properties is high, that value does not take into consideration the negative impact that heightened blood-sugar levels have on your waistline, skin, and health.

I'm certainly not against fruit; it's natural and delicious. However, I also can't suggest in good conscience that you simply exercise "moderation" without giving you a guide. That's why I created 15/6; it puts a measurable limit on the amount of sugar you consume in general, and also when it relates directly to the fruit in your diet.

If you enjoy eating fruit like me, then you'll notice right away that 15 grams of sugar does not allow a lot when it comes to fruit consumption. Often I limit myself to a handful of blueberries or blackberries in the evening as a treat. I find now that just a handful satisfies my sweet-tooth craving while providing an added boost of antioxidants to help fight free radicals and reduce oxidative stress.

You can still enjoy the flavor of fruit by using much smaller amounts to jazz up your foods. Try adding a few thin slices of pear to a green salad for a taste sensation. You will be surprised by how a little fruit will go a long way once you recondition your taste buds by eliminating the steady onslaught of excessive sugar.

The Anti-Aging Industry Treats the Symptoms, Not the Cause

I saw a commercial for Febreze recently that showed a perky mother cruising around the house, bottle of air freshener in hand, happily eliminating odors with a simple squeeze of the trigger. As she stood amidst the clutter of a stereotypical male teenager's bedroom, I

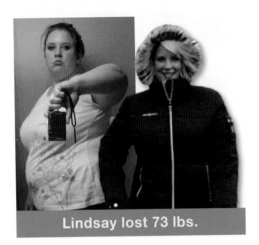

Lindsay lost 73 lbs.

Age: 33
Height: 5'7"
Belly Inches Lost: 15"

I gained 100 lbs. during my first pregnancy, but I believed all that weight would magically disappear after the birth of my child and with breast-feeding. That didn't happen! My unhealthy eating habits worsened as I adjusted to being a new mom. I felt hopeless. I lost some weight, but became pregnant again and gained more. The change finally came after I saw Jorge on *Rachael Ray*. I started his *The Aging Cure*™ plan the very next day.

At first, I felt like I was going through withdrawal; my body was so used to sugar. I had been consuming two McDonald's sweetened coffee drinks a day; I calculated those alone accounted for two weeks' worth of sugar! After two weeks, however, I had no trouble. I am so glad I found Jorge—I intend to eat *The Aging Cure*™ way for the rest of my life!

BEST TIP FOR SUCCESS:
I tell myself that tomorrow is always a new day, my next meal has new choices, and I never live in the past.

watched her unleash an animated mist over a hamper overflowing with dirty clothes with a satisfied smile on her face.

Problem solved, her expression suggested.

Wait a second, I thought. *She didn't solve the problem at all!*

In truth, the clothes needed to be run through the washer on Super Cycle, but she addressed the symptom of the unpleasant odor rather than the cause. I'd like to think she was only buying herself some time before the teen came home from football practice to have him take care of his dirty laundry. If not, she will return to that room every day—perhaps several times a day—to hide the odor again and again. The clothes will not stop smelling until they're cleaned.

In my opinion, so much of the anti-aging industry is like spraying Febreze on dirty clothes. We are offered a laundry list of supposed remedies to the visible effects of aging, but none of them address the true problem. That's why I tend to roll my eyes when I see a commercial for a topical cure all. In truth, moisturizers are only going after the symptoms. If you truly want to look younger, you must address the problem from the inside out.

The key is simple: my FAT-MELTING CARB SWAP™, which automatically avoids hidden sugar to prevent the formation of AGEs and keep your insulin levels balanced. I help you finally address the cause of the problem by showing you exactly what to eat to avoid hidden sugar and enjoy delicious, antioxidant-rich meals to promote healthy, flexible skin and look younger.

Younger-Looking You with a Smaller Waist

You only get one body. One life. In order to increase your quality *and* quantity life, you must get rid of the belly fat. That's my tough love for you, and I can say for certain that it's not your fault. You've been misinformed for a very long time, and I here to help you face the truth starting day.

Keep reading to learn additional benefits The Aging Cure™, and then commit to e of my easy-to-use One-Week Menus. vibrant new you is just around the corner!

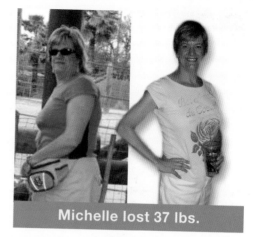

Michelle lost 37 lbs.

Age: 48
Height: 5'6"
Belly Inches Lost: 10"

At age 48, I was at my heaviest weight and realized I was on the verge of diabetes. I felt tired and sluggish all the time. I also suffered from acid reflux and severe headaches. After watching some of Jorge's videos on YouTube, I learned how dangerous sugar truly is. I decided to try The Aging Cure™. Right away, my acid reflux disappeared, and my headaches lessened. The weight melted off, and I found that I had more energy than ever before. My friends tell me I look ten years younger, and I *feel* ten years younger!

I want people to know that they too can lose the weight and feel like they're young again. This is not a diet—this is a lifestyle change for us all.

BEST TIP FOR SUCCESS:
Tell your friends your action plan to get started; making the commitment will help ensure you stay on track!

3 The One-Week Challenge
and Beyond

"Since losing weight with this program, I am lighter, brighter, and happier! Even though I am 63, I feel so much better than I felt when I was in my 30s and 40s. My energy is endless."

—BOBBI HALL, LOST 35 LBS.

This chapter is all about effortlessly applying the FAT-MELTING CARB SWAP™ to your life, starting today. *The Aging Cure*™ is a simple, revolutionary program to help you easily reverse visible signs of aging while dropping up to 9 lbs. every week. On the next few pages I tell you exactly what to eat to drop belly fat as well as look and feel younger in the next week.

I also recommend *The Aging Cure*™ as a lifestyle plan to increase your life span . . . however, I can't prove that to you in one week or even one year! This I do promise: if you stick to one of my easy-to-follow One-Week Menus, you will experience weight loss, look and feel younger, and position yourself to live well for years to come.

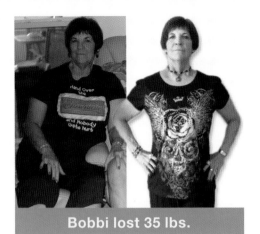

Bobbi lost 35 lbs.

Age: 63
Height: 5'3"
Belly Inches Lost: 5"

I was looking for a way to change my life for the better, not for a "Band-Aid" to cover up my problems. Because both of my parents had diabetes, a plan that focused on lowering the amounts of sugar and carbs in my diet appealed to me. I first discovered Jorge in *First for Women* magazine, and I started his program right away. After just three days, I lost weight and loved the way I felt, and I haven't stopped since.

Since losing weight with this program, I am lighter, brighter, and happier! I used to be unable to play with my granddaughters, but now they can't keep up with me! Even though I am 63, I feel so much better than I felt when I was in my 30s and 40s. My energy is endless, not only from eating foods that give me energy, but because of the joy I feel from looking so great.

BEST TIP FOR SUCCESS:
Do not approach this as a quick weight-loss method, but as a life change and as a preventive measure against obesity and illness. It's called a "cure" for a reason!

Your One-Week Menu

If you follow any of the menus in this chapter exactly, you'll begin a pattern of dietary health that will ultimately reduce your risk of disease to enhance both the quality and quantity of your life. You'll experience incredible weight-loss results as well as elevated energy and confidence. The benefits of your transformation will even benefit the loved ones around you. As your coach, I personally created this One-Week Menu and recipes to not only keep you on track, but for you to enjoy every bite and sip along the way.

You can absolutely continue to follow this simple plan after the first week and begin modifying your food options based on the magical and completely customizable formula of 15/6.

Right now, though, I want you to commit fully to following one of my One-Week Menus by signing the Success Contract the next page. I also recommend that you post this contract somewhere you can see it every day, as a reminder of your commitment to this program, to yourself, and those you care about.

The AGING CURE™

Agreement to Succeed

I commit fully to putting myself first by following 15/6 exactly in order to become a healthier, more confident person for myself and those I care about.

Current weight: _____

Goal weight 7 days from now: _____

Waist measurement*: _____

Goal waist measurement 7 days from now: _____

Your signature X_____

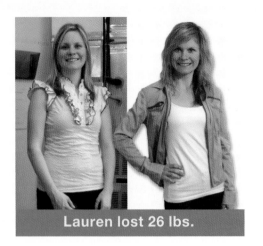

Lauren lost 26 lbs.

Age: 25
Height: 5'2"
Belly Inches Lost: 10"

I had never paid attention to what I ate. I constantly consumed processed food without even considering its effects on my body. I found that I felt tired all the time and knew I had to make a change. When I started *The Aging Cure*™, I became instantly hooked! Jorge's recipes were so easy, not to mention delicious. I now follow the plan all the time; it is that effective! Thanks to Jorge, I've changed my entire outlook on food . . . and on life!

BEST TIP FOR SUCCESS:
Always carry almonds and celery with you for a snack. That way you won't be compelled to eat an Age More food while out and about!

Getting Started

In order to get the best results, I recommend you follow one of the One-Week Menus exactly with no changes. I've done all the work to avoid confusion and build momentum instantly. Thousands of my clients have reached their goal weight and maintained a smaller waist long term by following my plan exactly. I highly recommend you model their success.

I understand that you might have personal preferences or dietary restrictions, however, so I designed these One-Week Menus to have flexibility. If you truly feel the need to make adjustments, there are five important guidelines to follow:

1. An entire day's menu can be repeated exactly every day for the entire week. For example, if Day 3 is your dream line-up, then repeat Day 3 for any other day, up to 7 days.

2. A meal or snack can be exchanged for another meal or snack within its same category from any day on the menu. For example, if dinner from Day 2 was incredible and you're ready to enjoy it for dinner again on Day 4 . . . you can! In the same way, a lunch can be exchanged for another lunch, and a snack for another snack.

3. Protein sources within a meal can be exchanged with your preferred protein sources. For example, if the protein for dinner is beef and you prefer chicken, feel free to have chicken instead.

4. Each of my One-Week Menus are all about easy, tossed-together meals. If, however, you love spending time in the kitchen, I've given you many tasty, FAT-MELTING CARB SWAP™ recipe options in Chapter 4 to substitute for lunch or dinner.

5. For those of you constantly on the go, I recommend substituting meals with a stevia-sweetened whey protein shake. Each shake should have at least 20 grams of protein and very low sugar (my personal recommendation is any shake from Jay Robb).

Quick Guidelines for Your One-Week Menu

- Before starting, take your preliminary waist measurement. Suck in your stomach and measure around your belly button. To determine your maximum healthy waist measurement, take your height and divide it in half. I am 6' tall (72") so I am aiming for a waist measurement less than 36". Go to JorgeCruise.com to watch Dr. Oz demonstrate exactly how to obtain an accurate measure.

- For those foods listed that do not have a serving size indicated, like chicken or beef, consider an amount equal to the size of your palm as a serving; eat no more than two servings of any one item in a sitting. Also, a palm-size serving and a heaping handful are not the same thing!

- Try to drink 6 to 8 glasses of water (48 to 64 fl. oz.) per day. If you need to urinate every 20 minutes, you may be overhydrated. If your urine is dark in color and/or cloudy, you are most likely dehydrated. Balance your hydration according to your thirst and the appearance of your urine.

- Yes, you may skip snacks or even meals if you're not physically hungry. But do not skip a snack or a meal if you *do* feel physically hungry.

Carb Lover's Menu

	DAY 1	DAY 2	DAY 3	DAY 4	DAY 5
BREAKFAST	1 English muffin topped with cream cheese and smoked salmon, served with 2 Tbsp. blueberries, and coffee with cream (5/2)	¼ cup steel-cut oats mixed with 2 Tbsp. walnuts and 2 Tbsp. blueberries, and coffee with cream (5/2)	2 scrambled eggs with cheddar cheese and 1 English muffin topped with butter, served with 2 Tbsp. blueberries, and coffee with cream (5/2)	¼ cup Ezekiel Food for Life Almond Cereal mixed with ½ cup unsweetened almond milk and 2 Tbsp. blueberries, and coffee with cream (4/2)	1 English muffin to with 2 slices Cana bacon, chedda cheese, and 1 fr egg; served with Tbsp. blueberries coffee with crea (5/2)
SNACK	1 hard-boiled egg (0/0)	1 handful almonds (0/0)	1 hard-boiled egg (0/0)	1 handful almonds (0/0)	1 hard-boiled e (0/0)
LUNCH	Deli turkey, spinach, ¼ cup salsa, and ¼ avocado wrapped in a whole-wheat tortilla; served with 5 tortilla chips (3/2)	Deli ham, ¼ cup sliced pickle, romaine, and mustard in half a whole-wheat pita (2/1)	¼ cup quinoa mixed with 2 Tbsp. peas and 2 Tbsp. chopped red pepper (4/2)	Deli turkey, 5 sliced cherry tomatoes, mozzarella, and romaine lettuce tossed in 2 Tbsp. creamy Caesar dressing; wrapped in a whole-wheat tortilla (3/2)	¼ cup chickpea Tbsp. chopped bell pepper, 2 T chopped red onio 2 Tbsp. cilantro mixed greens; tos olive oil and lime served with ½ to whole-wheat p (3/2)
SNACK	1 handful pumpkin seeds (0/0)	1 serving deli cheese (0/0)	1 handful pumpkin seeds (0/0)	1 serving deli cheese (0/0)	1 handfu pumpkin se (0/0)
DINNER	Whole-wheat pita topped with fresh mozzarella, ½ sliced tomato, and basil baked into a pizza (4/2)	2 oz. cooked whole-wheat penne mixed with pancetta, ricotta cheese, and basil (3/2)	Rotisserie chicken, spinach, and Parmesan cheese heated between 2 tortillas to make a quesadilla; served with ¼ cup Seeds of Change Tomato Basil Genovese sauce for dipping (1/2)	Whole-wheat pita topped with 2 Tbsp. Alfredo sauce, 2 Tbsp. chopped kalamata olives, 2 Tbsp. chopped red onion, 2 Tbsp. chopped sun-dried tomatoes, and a few torn basil leaves baked into a pizza (5/2)	2 oz. cooked wheat penne with choppe 3 chopped as spears, and fontina che (2/2)

DAY 6	DAY 7
¼ cup steel-cut oats mixed with 2 Tbsp. sliced almonds and 2 Tbsp. blueberries, and coffee with cream (5/2)	1 English muffin topped with cream cheese and 2 Tbsp. Nature's Hollow jam, with 2 sausage links; served with 2 Tbsp. blueberries, and coffee with cream (5/2)
1 handful almonds (0/0)	1 hard-boiled egg (0/0)
¼ cup quinoa mixed with 3 sliced strawberries and ricotta cheese (4/2)	Deli turkey, Swiss cheese, spinach, 3 tomato slices, and 2 Tbsp. hummus wrapped in a whole-wheat tortilla (2/2)
1 serving deli cheese (0/0)	1 handful pumpkin seeds (0/0)
Turkey, spinach, and mozzarella cheese heated between 2 tortillas to make a quesadilla; served with ¼ cup Seeds of Change Tomato Basil Genovese sauce for dipping (1/2)	Whole-wheat pita topped with mozzarella, pepperoni, 1 Tbsp. chopped onion, 1 Tbsp. chopped green bell pepper, and 2 Tbsp. sliced black olives baked into a pizza (4/2)

- Remember, dressings and sauces can make or break your weight loss. If you're considering making any swaps or additions to my plan, please carefully read the nutrition label for sugar and carbs.

- As your coach, let me again encourage you to stick to the program fully for one week. The results are incredible.

Day 8 and Beyond

After you complete the One-Week Menu, be sure to keep using one of the One-Week Menus with the FAT-MELTING CARB SWAP™ Recipes, and track your daily 15/6. This is how I live my life, and I don't regret it for a second. I've personally experienced the transformative results of this program, and I want the same for you.

Chicken and Seafood Menu

	DAY 1	DAY 2	DAY 3	DAY 4	DAY 5
BREAKFAST	2 poached eggs served atop a bed of sautéed spinach with 2 links chicken sausage, with 1 slice whole-wheat toast with butter, and coffee with cream (0/1)	2-egg omelette with turkey, spinach, and mozzarella cheese; with 1 slice whole-wheat toast with butter, and coffee with cream (0/1)	2 fried eggs served atop a bed of sautéed spinach and 2 links chicken sausage, with 1 slice whole-wheat toast with butter, and coffee with cream (0/1)	2-egg omelette with turkey, ½ cup broccoli, and cheddar cheese; with 1 slice whole-wheat toast with butter, and coffee with cream (1/1)	2 scrambled eg served atop a be spinach and 2 l chicken sausa with 1 slice wh wheat toast w butter, and cof with cream (0/1)
SNACK	1 handful walnuts (0/0)	1 handful macadamia nuts (0/0)	1 handful walnuts (0/0)	1 handful macadamia nuts (0/0)	1 handful waln (0/0)
LUNCH	Deli turkey, 5 sliced grapes, mozzarella, and romaine lettuce tossed in creamy Caesar dressing wrapped in a whole-wheat tortilla (5/1)	1 can salmon mixed with ¼ cup chopped red bell pepper and ¼ cup chopped cucumber tossed in olive oil in a whole-wheat pita (4/2)	Spinach topped with cooked shrimp, ½ sliced avocado, and ½ cup sliced cherry tomatoes tossed in lemon juice; served with ½ small sourdough roll with butter (4/2)	Rotisserie chicken mixed with ¼ cup blueberries and feta cheese on arugula tossed in 2 Tbsp. Italian dressing (5/1)	1 can tuna mix with mayo wi romaine lettu Muenster chee and ¼ toma wrapped in a to (3/1)
SNACK	1 string cheese stick (0/0)	1 serving deli turkey (0/0)	1 string cheese stick (0/0)	1 serving deli turkey (0/0)	1 string cheese (0/0)
DINNER	1 sliced grilled chicken breast, ½ avocado, and 5 halved cherry tomatoes tossed in olive oil and vinegar; served atop a bed of spinach (4/1)	1 turkey breast served with ½ cup broccoli, and 1 small slice of baguette with butter (2/2)	1 grilled chicken breast topped with 5 halved grape tomatoes, 5 halved kalamata olives, and feta cheese (3/1)	1 grilled salmon fillet with lemon juice, served with 3 spears asparagus and ½ cup brown rice (2/2)	1 grilled chic sandwich wit bun removed, with romaine, tomato, 2 sl bacon, and (3/2)

34

DAY 6	DAY 7
2-egg omelette with turkey, spinach, and feta cheese; with 1 slice whole-wheat toast with butter, and coffee with cream (0/1)	2 hard-boiled eggs served with a side of sautéed spinach and 2 links chicken sausage, with 1 slice whole-wheat toast with butter, and coffee with cream (0/1)
1 handful macadamia nuts (0/0)	1 handful walnuts (0/0)
1 turkey burger spread with mayo and topped with ½ avocado and 3 slices tomato, with ½ cup brown rice (3/2)	Rotisserie chicken atop a bed of spinach, with ½ cup chopped cucumber and crumbled blue cheese tossed in olive oil and vinegar (1/1)
1 serving deli turkey (0/0)	1 string cheese stick (0/0)
1 baked tilapia fillet topped with Parmesan cheese, served with a spinach salad tossed in oil and vinegar and topped with ¼ sliced avocado (1/1)	1 grilled chicken breast wrapped in sage leaves and prosciutto, topped with sautéed spinach; served with 1 small slice of baguette with butter (1/2)

Keep Your Sanity with Indulgent Snacks

I believe it's critical to enjoy what you eat in order to commit fully to one of the One-Week Menus as well as make *The Aging Cure*™ a lifestyle. Therefore, I've included dark chocolate in the Dessert Lover's Menu. I recommend chocolate with a cacao content of 85% or more, for a higher antioxidant content with the least amount of sugar. The best part is the taste, of course, but here's an added benefit: cacao contains bioflavonoids. The bioflavonoids in dark chocolate help you improve longevity, prevent disease, and maintain a youthful appearance.

Another favorite indulgence of mine is red wine. (Now, if you are not over 21 or if you're not a fan of wine, then obviously you can skip it and still experience the transformative results of *The Aging Cure*™.) Cabernet sauvignon is one of my go-to selections. Oftentimes I'll try to track down an organic option to avoid potential traces of pesticides and other added chemicals. Another health benefit to red wine is that it is full of resveratrol.

Faster Results Menu

	DAY 1	DAY 2	DAY 3	DAY 4	DAY 5
BREAKFAST	2 scrambled eggs with 2 Tbsp. salsa and cheddar cheese, and coffee with cream (1/1)	1 serving cottage cheese with ¼ cup chopped walnuts and 1 packet Truvia, and coffee with cream (3/1)	2-egg omelette with spinach and feta cheese, served with 2 links turkey bacon, and coffee with cream (0/0)	1 serving cottage cheese with 2 Tbsp. blueberries and 1 packet Truvia, and coffee with cream (5/1)	2 scrambled e with ham and S cheese, and co with cream (0/0)
SNACK	1 string cheese stick (0/0)	1 hard-boiled egg (0/0)	1 string cheese stick (0/0)	1 hard-boiled egg (0/0)	1 string cheese (0/0)
LUNCH	1 grilled chicken breast topped with 5 halved grape tomatoes, 5 halved kalamata olives, and feta cheese (3/1)	1 grilled tuna fillet served with cucumber slices topped with goat cheese (1/0)	Rotisserie chicken served atop a bed of spinach, with ½ cup chopped cucumber and feta tossed in olive oil and vinegar (1/0)	1 grilled salmon fillet atop arugula mixed with 2 Tbsp. chopped pecans and tossed in olive oil and vinegar (1/0)	1 sliced grill chicken breas cheese atop r greens tosse olive oil and vi dressing, serve 3 artichoke h (3/1)
SNACK	3 slices salami (0/0)	1 handful olives (0/0)	3 slices salami (0/0)	1 handful olives (0/0)	3 slices sal (0/0)
DINNER	Steak with ½ cup mashed cauliflower with butter, and 3 grilled asparagus spears topped with Parmesan cheese (3/1)	1 sautéed pork loin served with ¼ cup mushrooms and ¼ cup squash (1/1)	2 hamburger patties topped with 3 slices tomato, mayo, and mustard; wrapped in lettuce (2/1)	1 grilled tilapia fillet served with ¼ cup chopped broccoli and ¼ cup chopped cauliflower (1/1)	1 turkey b spread with and toppec spinach and tomato, se with ½ cup s brussels sp (3/1)

DAY 6	DAY 7
1 serving cottage cheese with ¼ cup sliced almonds and 1 packet Truvia, and coffee with cream (3/1)	2-egg omelette with 3 slices tomato and basil, with 2 links sausage, and coffee with cream (0/0)
1 hard-boiled egg (0/0)	1 string cheese stick (0/0)
Spinach topped with cooked shrimp, ½ sliced avocado, and ½ cup sliced cherry tomatoes tossed in lemon juice (3/1)	Rotisserie chicken served atop spinach tossed in olive oil and vinegar, served with ½ cup sliced zucchini (1/0)
1 handful olives (0/0)	3 slices salami (0/0)
1 sautéed halibut fillet served with ¼ cup chopped cauliflower and ¼ cup chopped artichoke hearts (2/1)	1 hamburger patty topped with a fried egg, served with ½ cup cucumber slices (1/0)

My friend Dr. Oz is a proponent of this substance to increase vitality and for its anti-aging properties.

If you prefer white wine, that is absolutely allowed on The Aging Cure™ as well. It typically boasts an S/C Value of 0/0, which is perfect. However, it doesn't have the added benefit of the resveratrol because that comes from grape skins, which are not used when fermenting white wine (as opposed to red wine).

Again, I want you to enjoy what you're eating as you drop all the belly fat. That's why I created The Aging Cure™ to be both delicious and completely satisfying. Cheers!

Meat Madness Menu

	DAY 1	DAY 2	DAY 3	DAY 4	DAY 5
BREAKFAST	2-egg omelette with ham, ¼ cup chopped broccoli florets, and cheddar cheese; served with 2 strips bacon, and coffee with cream (1/0)	2 scrambled eggs with sausage and Swiss cheese, and coffee with cream (0/0)	2-egg omelette with spinach and feta cheese, served with 2 links chicken sausage, and coffee with cream (0/0)	2 scrambled eggs with hot sauce and cheddar cheese, with 2 slices Canadian bacon, and coffee with cream (1/1)	2-egg omelette 3 slices tomato basil, with 2 li sausage, and c with cream (0/0)
SNACK	1 handful sunflower seeds (0/0)	1 handful peanuts (0/0)	1 handful sunflower seeds (0/0)	1 handful peanuts (0/0)	1 handful sunflower see (0/0)
LUNCH	Roast beef, provolone cheese, ½ cup chopped broccoli florets, and horseradish mustard wrapped in a whole-wheat tortilla served with a handful of Pirate's Booty (2/2)	Deli turkey, 5 sliced cherry tomatoes, mozzarella, and romaine lettuce tossed in 2 Tbsp. creamy Caesar dressing; wrapped in a whole-wheat tortilla (3/2)	1 grilled hamburger patty covered in ½ cup Seeds of Change Marinara, served atop a bed of spinach (0/1)	Deli ham, ¼ cup sliced pickle, romaine, and mustard in ½ a whole-wheat pita (2/1)	Roast beef, chee cheese, 3 slice tomato, and rom lettuce; served o slices Ezekiel Fo for Life 4:9 Sprou 100% Whole Gr Bread spread w mustard and ma (2/2)
SNACK	1 hard-boiled egg (0/0)	1 handful olives (0/0)	1 hard-boiled egg (0/0)	1 handful olives (0/0)	1 hard-boiled eg (0/0)
DINNER	Steak cooked in olive oil and garlic, served with 5 steak fries and 2 Tbsp. Nature's Hollow Sugar-Free Ketchup (2/2)	1 turkey breast served with ½ cup mashed potatoes with butter and ½ cup squash (2/2)	½ lb. flank steak, 2 Tbsp. salsa, and 2 Tbsp. chopped avocado in a whole-wheat tortilla served with ¼ cup brown rice (5/2)	1 grilled chicken sandwich with top bun removed, topped with romaine, 3 slices tomato, 2 slices bacon, and mayo (3/2)	Steak cooked in o oil, served with ½ c mashed potatoes v butter, and 3 grille asparagus spear topped with Parme (5/2)

DAY 6	DAY 7
2 scrambled eggs with tomato and basil, with 2 links chicken sausage, and coffee with cream (2/1)	2-egg omelette with 2 Tbsp. chopped onion and garlic, and 2 slices bacon, and coffee with cream (1/0)
1 handful peanuts (0/0)	1 handful sunflower seeds (0/0)
Deli turkey, Swiss cheese, spinach, 3 tomato slices, and 2 Tbsp. hummus; wrapped in a whole-wheat tortilla (2/2)	3 meatballs topped with ¼ cup Seeds of Change marinara sauce, with a side Caesar salad of romaine lettuce, Parmesan cheese, ¼ cup croutons, and 2 Tbsp. Caesar dressing (2/1)
1 handful olives (0/0)	1 hard-boiled egg (0/0)
1 grilled chicken breast with goat cheese, atop mixed greens tossed in olive oil and vinegar dressing; served with artichoke (1/1)	½ lb. flank steak, 2 Tbsp. salsa, and 2 Tbsp. chopped avocado in a whole-wheat tortilla; served with ¼ cup brown rice (5/2)

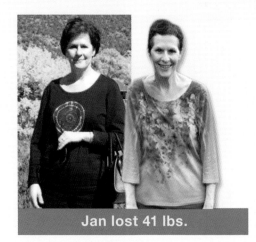

Jan lost 41 lbs.

Age: 62
Height: 5'6"
Belly Inches Lost: 11"

After a hip replacement at age 57, I wanted to look better and feel better about myself. I had read about Jorge in the *Costco Connection* magazine, so I decided to give his program a try. From the very first day I began *The Aging Cure*™, I was *never* hungry! Before I knew it, I had dropped 20 lbs., but I didn't stop there. I am now at 125 lbs.—which is how much I weighed as a teenager! I absolutely love my new life, and I have begun inspiring others to do this program as well.

BEST TIP FOR SUCCESS:
Always bring a snack.
I love bringing cheese with
me if I know I'm going to be
in a pinch.

Quick and Easy Menu

	DAY 1	DAY 2	DAY 3	DAY 4	DAY 5
BREAKFAST	Starbucks Perfect Oatmeal with Nut Medley, and coffee with cream (0/2)	McDonald's Sausage Burrito, and coffee with cream (2/2)	Burger King Sausage Burrito, and coffee with cream (2/2)	Starbucks Spinach & Feta Breakfast Wrap, and coffee with cream (4/2)	McDonald's Sausa Burrito, and coffe with cream (2/2)
SNACK	1 scoop chocolate Jay Robb whey protein mixed with water (0/0)	1 string cheese stick (0/0)	1 scoop chocolate Jay Robb whey protein mixed with water (0/0)	1 string cheese stick (0/0)	1 scoop chocola Jay Robb whey pr mixed with wat (0/0)
LUNCH	Quiznos large Mediterranean Chicken Salad (5/1)	Starbucks Tuna Salad Bistro Box (4/2)	Lean Cuisine Broccoli Cheddar Dip with Pita Bread (4/2)	Starbucks Chicken & Hummus Bistro Box (4/2)	Panera Bread Chopped Chick Cobb with Avoc (3/1)
SNACK	1 handful almonds (0/0)	1 handful sunflower seeds (0/0)	1 handful almonds (0/0)	1 handful sunflower seeds (0/0)	1 handful almo (0/0)
DINNER	⅓ Amy's Margherita Pizza (3/2)	Stouffer's Beef Stroganoff (4/2)	Smart Ones Chicken & Broccoli Alfredo (1/2)	Amy's Light & Lean Pasta & Veggies (3/2)	Lean Cuisi Rosemary Ch (5/2)

DAY 6	DAY 7
Burger King Sausage Burrito, and coffee with cream (2/2)	Starbucks Perfect Oatmeal with Nut Medley, and coffee with cream (0/2)
1 string cheese stick (0/0)	1 scoop chocolate Jay Robb whey protein mixed with water (0/0)
Starbucks Chipotle Chicken Wrap (5/2)	Smart Ones Three Cheese and Black Bean Quesadilla (3/2)
1 handful sunflower seeds (0/0)	1 handful almonds (0/0)
Stouffer's Green Pepper Steak (5/2)	⅓ Kashi Thin Crust Basil Pesto Pizza (2/2)

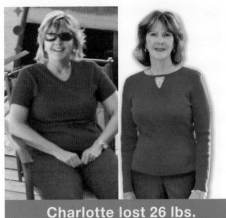

Charlotte lost 26 lbs.

Age: 55
Height: 5'6"
Belly Inches Lost: 9"

I saw a friend of mine at church wearing a form-fitting turquoise dress. She had lost weight thanks to Jorge Cruise and looked fabulous. I wondered if I could achieve the same results.

I gave her several excuses as to why I couldn't lose the weight—I'm too old, I'm menopausal, I've tried before—but she believed in me and encouraged me to try. I'm so thankful for her encouragement. The weight started coming off right away. I even stayed on the program when I traveled to Hong Kong; it's that easy. When my husband and I traveled to Cabo San Lucas over three years ago, I was a size 16. I'm happy to say that when I return this year I will be a size 8! My friend is even loaning me her gorgeous turquoise dress to wear on the trip.

BEST TIP FOR SUCCESS:
Write down everything from Day One— weight, what you have to eat, exercise. That way you can really see how much you've progressed, and it will motivate you to continue!

Dessert Lover's Menu

	DAY 1	DAY 2	DAY 3	DAY 4	DAY 5
BREAKFAST	2 scrambled eggs with 2 Tbsp. salsa and cheddar cheese, and coffee with cream (1/0)	2-egg omelette with spinach and feta cheese, served with 2 links chicken sausage, and coffee with cream (0/0)	1 scoop chocolate Jay Robb whey protein mixed with water (0/0)	2 scrambled eggs with 2 Tbsp. hot sauce and cheddar cheese, and coffee with cream (0/0)	2-egg omelette ham, 3 slices to and mozzare cheese; and co with cream (0/0)
LUNCH	Romaine lettuce topped with cooked shrimp, ½ sliced avocado, and ½ cup sliced cherry tomatoes tossed in lemon juice (3/1)	Deli turkey, 5 sliced cherry tomatoes, mozzarella, and romaine lettuce tossed in 2 Tbsp. creamy Caesar dressing; wrapped in a whole-wheat tortilla (3/2)	1 grilled hamburger patty topped with romaine lettuce, 3 tomato slices, 2 slices bacon, cheddar cheese, mustard, and mayo (3/1)	1 grilled salmon fillet, atop arugula mixed with 2 Tbsp. chopped walnuts and tossed in olive oil and vinegar (1/0)	Deli turkey, Sw cheese, spinach tomato slices, a 2 Tbsp. humm wrapped in a wh wheat tortilla (2/2)
SNACK	1 hard-boiled egg (0/0)	1 string cheese stick (0/0)	1 hard-boiled egg (0/0)	1 string cheese stick (0/0)	1 hard-boiled eg (0/0)
DINNER	1 grilled chicken breast topped with romaine, 3 slices tomato, 2 slices bacon, and mayo (3/0)	Rotisserie chicken, spinach, and feta cheese heated between 2 tortillas to make a quesadilla; served with ¼ cup Seeds of Change Tomato Basil Genovese sauce for dipping (1/2)	Steak cooked in olive oil and garlic, served with ½ cup chopped broccoli florets topped with melted cheddar cheese (1/1)	1 grilled chicken breast topped with 5 halved grape tomatoes, 5 halved kalamata olives, and feta cheese (3/1)	Rotisserie chicke chopped brocco florets, and chedd cheese heated between 2 tortillas make a quesadilla served with ¼ cup Seeds of Change Tomato Basil Genov sauce for dipping (1/2)
TREAT	¼ cup Clemmy's Chocolate Ice Cream (0/2)	12 pieces Green & Black's Dark 85% Chocolate (5/1)	¼ cup Clemmy's Chocolate Ice Cream (0/2)	12 pieces Green & Black's Dark 85% Chocolate (5/1)	¼ cup Clemmy's Chocolate Ice Crea (0/2)

DAY 6	DAY 7
1 scoop chocolate Jay Robb whey protein mixed with water (0/0)	2 scrambled eggs with 2 Tbsp. salsa and cheddar cheese, and coffee with cream (1/0)
1 grilled turkey burger covered in ½ cup Seeds of Change Marinara served atop a bed of spinach (0/1)	1 can tuna mixed with mayo, mixed with Romaine lettuce, cheddar cheese, and ¼ sliced tomato (3/1)
1 string cheese stick (0/0)	1 hard-boiled egg (0/0)
Steak cooked in olive oil served with ½ cup mashed potatoes with butter, and 3 grilled asparagus spears topped with Parmesan (5/2)	1 grilled chicken breast topped with creamy goat cheese, served with sautéed spinach (0/0)
12 pieces Green & Black's Dark 85% Chocolate (5/1)	¼ cup Clemmy's Chocolate Ice Cream (0/2)

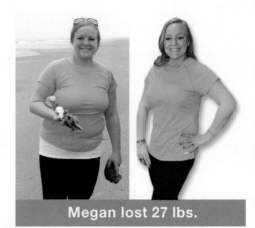

Megan lost 27 lbs.

Age: 24
Height: 5'2"
Belly Inches Lost: 6.5"

After noticing how great my aunt looked on a trip to the beach, I asked her how she had lost the weight. When she told me about the Jorge's recommendations, I was skeptical. She was eating delicious food throughout the whole trip; how could she be losing weight? I started *The Aging Cure*™ when I returned from the trip and gave it a try. I lost 6 lbs. in just the first week! I couldn't believe it. I wasn't starving and was enjoying what I ate. I have now gone from a size 14 to a size 8. I'm so thankful that my aunt introduced me to Jorge. He has truly changed my life forever!

BEST TIP FOR SUCCESS:
Enjoy your food—
make every meal something
you look forward to!

Vegan/Vegetarian Menu

	DAY 1	DAY 2	DAY 3	DAY 4	DAY 5
BREAKFAST	1 English muffin topped with 2 Tbsp. Nature's Hollow Sugar-Free Strawberry Preserves, and coffee with 2 Tbsp. unsweetened almond milk (1/2)	¼ cup steel-cut oats mixed with 2 Tbsp. chopped walnuts and 2 Tbsp. blueberries, and coffee with 2 Tbsp. unsweetened almond milk (3/2)	1 English muffin topped with 2 Tbsp. almond butter, and coffee with 2 Tbsp. unsweetened almond milk (3/2)	¼ cup Ezekiel Food for Life Almond Cereal mixed with ½ cup unsweetened almond milk and 2 Tbsp. blueberries, and coffee with 2 Tbsp. unsweetened almond milk (3/2)	1 English muffin topped with 2 Tbsp. Nature's Hollow Sugar-Free Apricot Preserve and coffee with 2 Tbsp. unsweetened almond milk (1/2)
SNACK	1 handful pistachios (0/0)	1 handful macadamia nuts (0/0)	1 handful pistachios (0/0)	1 handful macadamia nuts (0/0)	1 handful pistachios (0/0)
LUNCH	Sautéed artichoke hearts and ¼ avocado, atop a bed of arugula tossed in olive oil and vinegar; served with ½ cup brown rice (2/2)	¼ cup chickpeas, 2 Tbsp. chopped red bell pepper, 2 Tbsp. chopped red onion, and 2 Tbsp. cilantro over mixed greens tossed in olive oil and lime juice; served with ½ toasted whole-wheat pita (3/2)	½ cup mushrooms sautéed in garlic and spinach, stuffed in a whole-wheat pita (2/2)	¼ cup black beans, ¼ cup canned corn, 2 Tbsp. chopped tomato, 2 Tbsp. chopped onion, 2 Tbsp. cilantro over romaine tossed in vegan ranch dressing (4/2)	¼ baked sweet potato served with ½ cup brussels sprouts (5/1)
SNACK	1 handful olives (0/0)	1 handful sunflower seeds (0/0)	1 handful olives (0/0)	1 handful sunflower seeds (0/0)	1 handful olives (0/0)
DINNER	1 veggie patty topped with mayo and 3 slices of tomato, served with ½ cup sliced cucumber (3/1)	½ cup sliced cooked eggplant, ½ cup sliced cooked zucchini, and 2 Tbsp. chopped parsley cooked in garlic; served with ½ cup Seeds of Change marinara (3/1)	Tofu cooked in ½ cup Seeds of Change marinara, with spinach and 2 Tbsp. chopped walnuts (1/1)	2 oz. whole-wheat linguine mixed with ½ cup chopped broccoli, 2 Tbsp. chopped tomatoes, and 1 Tbsp. butter (2/1)	1 veggie patty topped with mustard and 3 slices tomato wrapped in romaine leaves, served with 5 steak fries and 2 Tbsp. Nature's Hollow Sugar-Free ketchup (3/2)

DAY 6	DAY 7
¼ cup steel-cut oats mixed with 2 Tbsp. sliced almonds and 2 Tbsp. blueberries, and coffee with 2 Tbsp. unsweetened almond milk (3/2)	1 English muffin topped with 2 Tbsp. hummus, and coffee with 2 Tbsp. unsweetened almond milk (1/2)
1 handful macadamia nuts (0/0)	1 handful pistachios (0/0)
¼ cup white beans mixed with 2 Tbsp. chopped roasted red pepper over a bed of spinach, served with 5 pita chips (2/2)	¼ cup quinoa mixed with 2 Tbsp. peas and 2 Tbsp. chopped red bell pepper (4/2)
1 handful sunflower seeds (0/0)	1 handful olives (0/0)
1 whole-wheat pita topped with ¼ cup pesto, 2 Tbsp. sliced black olives, 2 Tbsp. chopped red onion, and 2 Tbsp. chopped green bell pepper (5/2)	Tofu cooked in garlic served atop a bed of spinach tossed with olive oil (0/0)

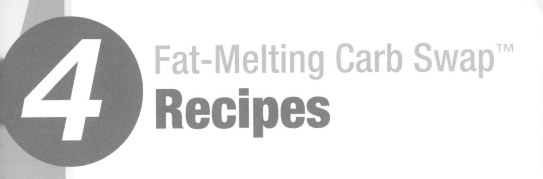

Fat-Melting Carb Swap™
Recipes

I genuinely believe that the cure for aging begins in the kitchen, and it's time for you to eat delicious, antioxidant-rich meals that reverse, rather than accelerate, the signs of aging. From aromatic herbs like rosemary and thyme to powerful spices like peppercorns and cinnamon, I've snuck antioxidants into each dish that not only taste amazing, but as an added bonus, they improve your health! In this chapter you will uncover dozens of my favorite, all-new Age Less recipes that are low in hidden sugar and high in antioxidants (plus high in flavor!) to help you look young, feel young, and finally experience a smaller waist for life.

Note that each recipe included here has an S/C Value of 5/2 or less, so you can mix and match any of these meals and stay on track for 15/6 every day. Also, almost all of the following recipes serve four people. This is because they are so delicious that you'll want to serve them to your entire family—or have leftovers for the next day! And if a recipe says to season "to taste," you may season freely to your liking.

I encourage you to get creative with these recipes. Don't let a hard-to-find item or brand stop you from whipping up a dish. For example, if you can't find the pita bread I recommend, use another brand of pita with a low S/C Value.

Everyone's tastes are different, but I guarantee you're going to find something you love here. You'll soon forget that you're cooking for your health, and not just for your taste buds.

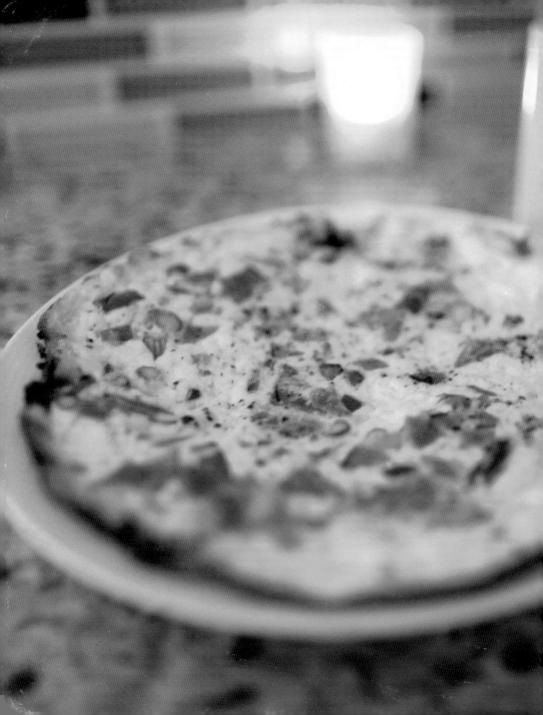

SHARP CHEDDAR HAM FRITTATA

SERVES 4

Antioxidants: onion, chives, asparagus, extra-virgin olive oil, black pepper, mixed greens

S/C Value = 0/0

Tbsp. onion, chopped

Tbsp. extra-virgin olive oil

eggs

Tbsp. half-and-half

cup sharp cheddar cheese, grated

cup ham, chopped

Tbsp. fresh chives, chopped

asparagus stalks, cut into 1" pieces

cups mixed greens

salt and pepper, to taste

. For frittata: Preheat oven to broil. Cook onion in 2 Tbsp. olive oil in an ovenproof skillet or a few minutes, or until barely softened. In a medium-sized bowl, whisk eggs, and add alf-and-half and cheese. Pour egg-and-cheese mixture into skillet, and season with salt nd pepper. Top with ham, chives, and asparagus. Turn heat to low and cook to seal bottom, bout 2 or 3 minutes. Place skillet under broiler and cook for 2 minutes, or until puffed and ust barely set. Remove from oven and let cool.

. For mixed greens: Place greens a large salad bowl. Toss with 1 Tbsp. olive oil. Season vith salt and pepper, to taste.

. Slice frittata into 4 pieces, and serve each with a side of mixed greens.

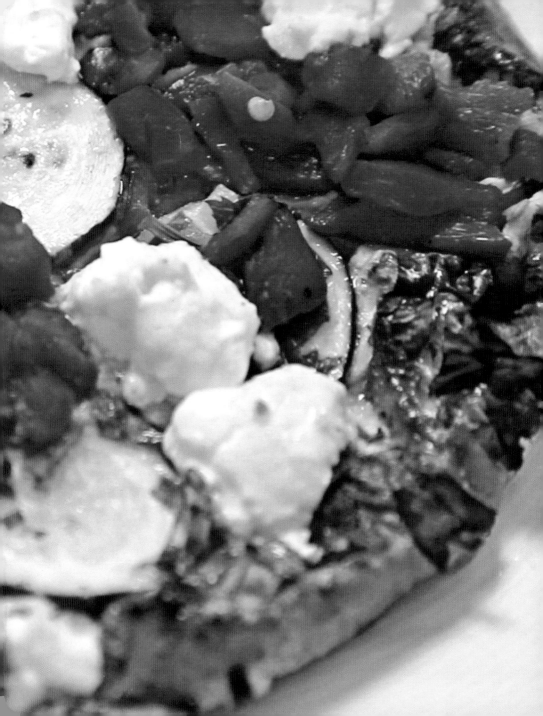

GOAT CHEESE AND ZUCCHINI FRITTATA

SERVES 4

Antioxidants: red onion, parsley, chives, extra-virgin olive oil, red peppers, black pepper

S/C Value = 0/0

¼ cup red onion, chopped
2 medium zucchini, thinly sliced
2 Tbsp. extra-virgin olive oil
8 eggs
Handful of fresh parsley, chopped
Handful of fresh chives, chopped
4 oz. fresh goat cheese
4 roasted red peppers, chopped
Salt and pepper, to taste

1. Preheat oven to broil. Cook onion and zucchini in olive oil in an ovenproof skillet for a few minutes, or until barely softened. In a medium-sized bowl, whisk eggs, and add parsley and chives. Pour egg into skillet; season with salt and pepper. Turn heat to low and cook for 2–3 minutes, or until the bottom of frittata is sealed. Top with goat cheese and roasted red peppers. Place under broiler for 2–3 minutes, until set. Remove from oven and let cool.

2. Cut frittata into 4 pieces and serve.

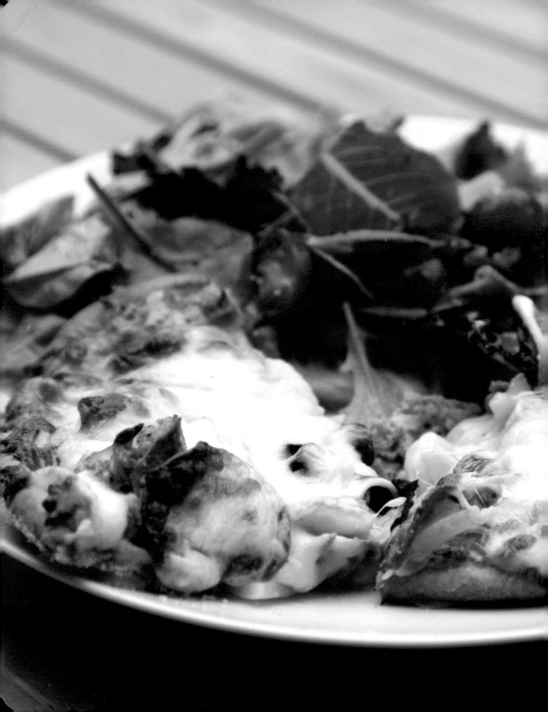

CHEESY SUPREME PIZZA

SERVES 2

Antioxidants: onion, olives, extra-virgin olive oil, black pepper, tomatoes, mixed greens, bell pepper

S/C Value = 5/2

Pizza:
oz. premade pizza dough
sausage links
flour, for preparing crust
Cornmeal, for preparing crust
½ cup pizza sauce
½ cup mozzarella cheese, grated
slices pepperoni
Tbsp. onion, chopped
Tbsp. green bell pepper, chopped
¼ cup black olives, drained
Tbsp. extra-virgin olive oil

Salad:
2 cups mixed greens
10 cherry tomatoes, sliced into halves
½ cup Parmesan cheese
Blue cheese dressing, for serving
Salt and pepper, to taste

1. Preheat oven to 425° F. Warm pizza stone* in oven for 20 minutes until hot. Cook sausage in olive oil in a skillet on low heat for 5 minutes, or until just cooked through. Move sausage from skillet to cutting board, allow to cool slightly, then slice. Roll 4 oz. ball of premade dough flat and very thin on a lightly floured surface. Sprinkle cornmeal on pizza peel* and place dough onto peel. Slide dough onto pizza stone in oven and precook for 3 minutes. Remove pizza from oven with peel and spread sauce onto crust. Top with mozzarella, meat, and veggies. Cook about 20 minutes, or until desired crispness. Remove pizza from oven with peel, and let cool slightly.

2. For salad: Mix greens, cherry tomatoes, and Parmesan in a large salad bowl. Toss with dressing and season with salt and pepper, to taste.

3. Slice pizza into 4 pieces, and serve 2 slices per person with a side of salad.

Note: If you do not have a pizza peel or pizza stone, you can use a baking sheet. Lightly sprinkle with cornmeal. Then place the rolled dough onto it, and follow the rest of the directions.

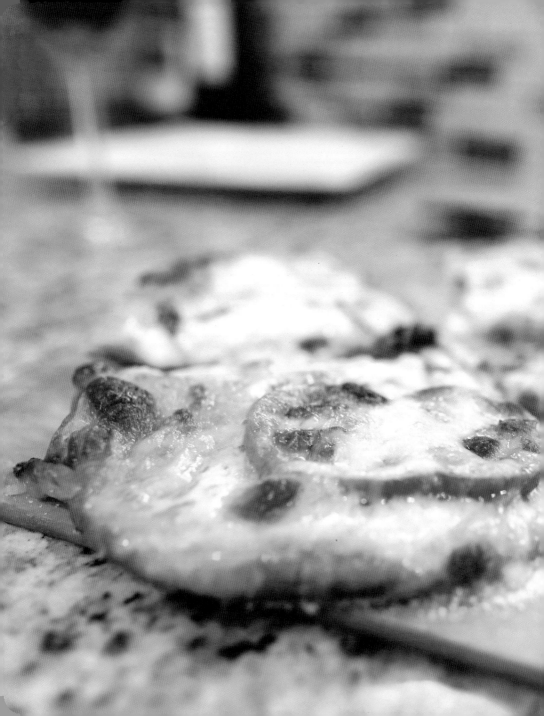

PERFECT MARGHERITA PIZZA

SERVES 2

Antioxidants: tomato, basil, extra-virgin olive oil

S/C Value = 3/2

4 oz. premade pizza dough
Flour, for preparing crust
Cornmeal, for preparing crust
1 tomato, thinly sliced
3 oz. fresh mozzarella, sliced
¼ cup fresh basil
1 Tbsp. extra-virgin olive oil

1. Preheat oven to 425° F. Warm pizza stone* in oven for 20 minutes until hot. Roll 4 oz. ball of premade dough flat and very thin on a lightly floured surface. Sprinkle cornmeal on pizza peel* and place dough onto peel. Slide dough onto pizza stone in oven and precook for 3 minutes. Pat dry tomatoes and mozzarella. Remove pizza from oven with peel. Arrange tomatoes and basil on pizza. Cover with mozzarella, then drizzle with olive oil. Cook for desired crispness (about 20 minutes). Remove pizza from oven with peel, and let cool slightly.

2. Slice into 4 pieces, and serve 2 slices for each person.

*Note: If you do not have a pizza peel or pizza stone, you can use a baking sheet. Lightly sprinkle with cornmeal. Then place the rolled dough onto it, and follow the rest of the directions.

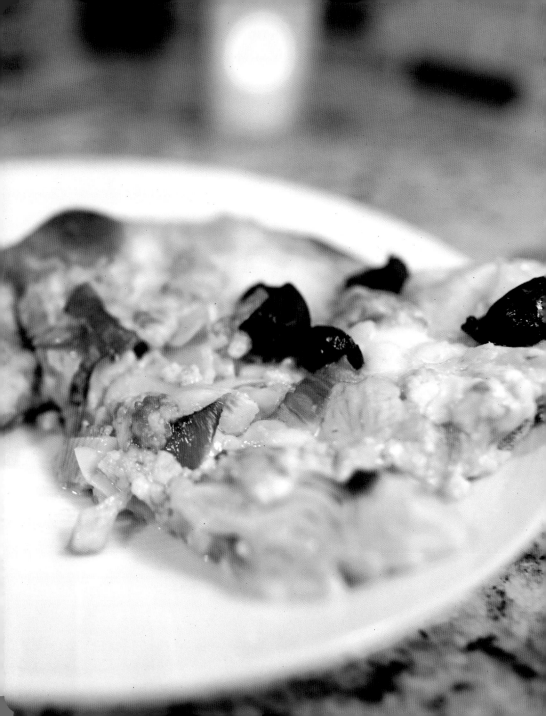

ARTICHOKE, ONION, AND OLIVE PIZZA

SERVES 2

Antioxidants: red onion, olives, artichoke hearts.

S/C Value = 3/2

4 oz. premade pizza dough

Flour, for preparing crust

Cornmeal, for preparing crust

1/2 cup blue cheese, crumbled

3 oz. fresh mozzarella cheese, sliced

1/2 red onion, sliced

1/2 cup olives, chopped

15 oz. canned artichoke hearts, drained and chopped

1. Preheat oven to 425° F. Warm pizza stone* in oven for 20 minutes until hot. Roll 4 oz. ball of premade dough flat and very thin on a lightly floured surface. Sprinkle cornmeal on pizza peel* and place dough onto peel. Slide dough onto pizza stone in oven and precook for 3 minutes. Remove pizza from oven with peel and place both cheeses on crust. Top with red onion, olives, and artichoke hearts. Cook for desired crispness (about 20 minutes). Remove pizza from oven with peel, and let cool slightly.

2. Slice into 4 pieces, and serve 2 slices for each person.

Note: If you do not have a pizza peel or pizza stone, you can use a baking sheet. Lightly sprinkle with cornmeal. Then place the rolled dough onto it, and follow the rest of the directions.

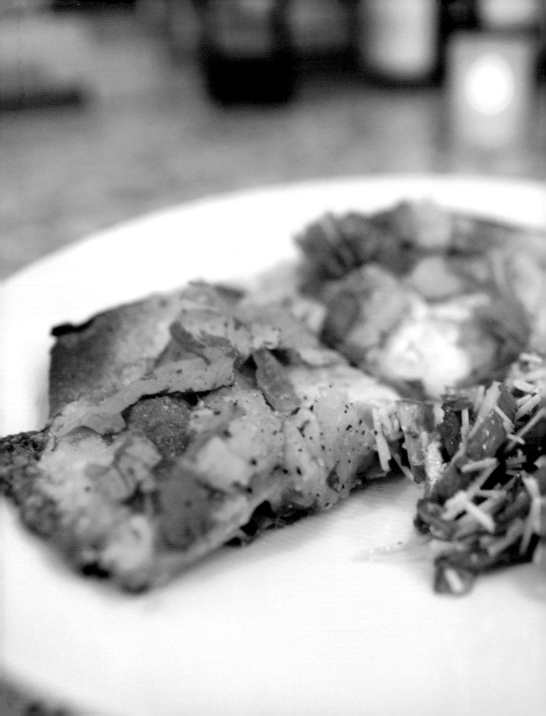

SWEET AND SAVORY GORGONZOLA PIZZA

SERVES 2

Antioxidants: extra-virgin olive oil, black pepper, arugula, lemon juice, parsley, squash, mushrooms

S/C Value = 5/2

Pizza:

½ lb. acorn squash
2 Tbsp. Nature's Hollow Maple
   Sugar-Free Syrup
1 tsp. red pepper flakes
Flour, for preparing crust
Cornmeal, for preparing crust
1 cup mozzarella, shredded
½ cup Gorgonzola, crumbled
1 cup arugula, torn in bite-size pieces
4 oz. premade pizza dough
1 Tbsp. extra-virgin olive oil
½ tsp. salt
½ tsp. pepper

Fresh Mushroom and Parsley Salad:

½ lb. large button mushrooms, sliced
¼ cup extra-virgin olive oil
¼ cup lemon juice
⅓ cup fresh parsley, chopped
Parmesan cheese, for serving
Salt and pepper, to taste

1. For pizza: Preheat oven to 375° F. Warm pizza stone* in oven for 20 minutes until hot. Slice squash in half from top to bottom; scoop out the seeds. Chop squash into ½"- and ¾"-wide half moons, and place in a medium bowl. Toss squash with syrup, olive oil, red pepper flakes, ¼ tsp. salt, and ¼ tsp. pepper. Place the squash on a parchment-lined baking sheet, and bake until tender and golden (about 20–25 minutes). Remove from oven and turn oven to 425°. Roll 4 oz. ball of premade dough flat and very thin on a lightly floured surface. Sprinkle cornmeal on pizza peel* and place dough onto peel. Slide dough onto pizza stone in oven and precook for 3 minutes. Remove pizza from oven with peel. Sprinkle the mozzarella cheese and the Gorgonzola onto pizza. Cook for desired crispness (about 20 minutes). Peel skins off squash. Remove pizza from oven with peel, and top with cooked squash. Top with arugula and ¼ tsp. salt and ¼ tsp. pepper.

2. For salad: Whisk together olive oil and lemon juice until smooth. Season with salt and pepper, to taste. Add mushrooms and parsley and toss to coat. Top with Parmesan cheese.

3. Slice pizza into 4 pieces, and serve 2 slices per person with a side of salad.

*Note: If you do not have a pizza peel or pizza stone, you can use a baking sheet. Lightly sprinkle with cornmeal. Then place the rolled dough onto it, and follow the rest of the directions.

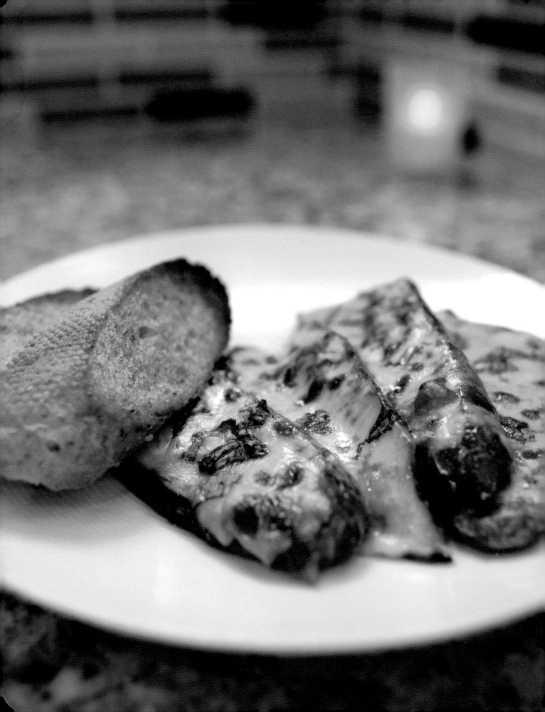

CHEESY PIZZA STRIPS

SERVES 4

Antioxidants: basil, extra-virgin olive oil, black pepper, garlic

S/C Value = 4/1

Pizza strips:

2 cucumbers

1/2 cup Seeds of Change Tomato
Basil Genovese Pasta Sauce

1 cup mozzarella, grated

4 fresh basil leaves, chopped

Extra-virgin olive oil, as needed

Salt and pepper, to taste

Garlic toast:

8" baguette, cut into 4 portions

1 garlic clove, sliced into 2 pieces

Extra-virgin olive oil

1. Preheat oven to broil. Slice each cucumber in half lengthwise, then cut each half into thirds lengthwise, for a total of 12 long strips. Brush each side of cucumber with olive oil; season with salt and pepper, to taste. Place on a baking sheet lined with aluminum foil, and broil for 1 minute on each side. Top with sauce, mozzarella, and basil; broil for an additional minute.

2. For garlic toast: Brush each slice of baguette with olive oil and rub garlic clove onto them. Place under broiler for 3 minutes, or until golden.

3. Serve cucumber strips warm, with a slice of garlic toast.

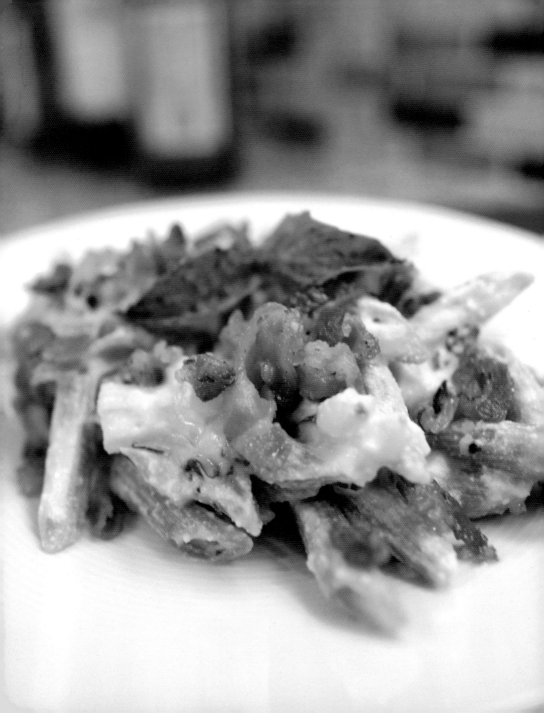

PANCETTA PENNE

SERVES 4

Antioxidants: onion, basil, extra-virgin olive oil, black pepper

S/C Value = 3/2

7 oz. whole-wheat penne pasta
3 slices pancetta
½ large onion, sliced
1 cup ricotta cheese, at room temperature
5 fresh basil leaves, chopped
1 Tbsp. extra-virgin olive oil
Salt and pepper, to taste

1. In a large pot of boiling salted water, cook the penne according to directions on packaging; set aside. Cook pancetta in olive oil in a skillet until crisp, and transfer to a plate. Add the onions to the skillet and cook until golden (about 10 minutes). Stir the onions and ricotta into the pasta, followed by the basil. Season with salt and pepper, to taste.

2. Crumble the pancetta and sprinkle it over the pasta before serving.

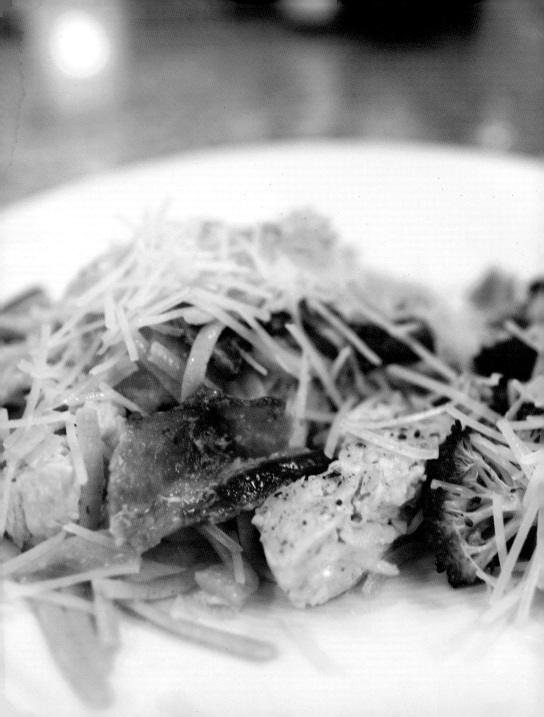

ZESTY CHICKEN BACON LINGUINE

SERVES 4

Antioxidants: onion, black pepper, broccoli, garlic, extra-virgin olive oil

S/C Value = 3/2

Linguine:

6 oz. linguine

12 oz. bacon, chopped

2 chicken breasts

1 Tbsp. extra-virgin olive oil

1 large onion, thinly sliced

2 egg yolks

Parmesan cheese, for serving

Salt and pepper, to taste

Broccoli:

1 head broccoli, chopped into tiny florets

¼ cup Parmesan cheese, grated

2 garlic cloves, minced

Salt and pepper, to taste

1 Tbsp. extra-virgin olive oil

1. For linguine: Place chicken breasts on a flat surface, lay a sheet of plastic wrap over them, and pound flat with a mallet. Cook chicken in olive oil in a skillet over medium heat for 5–8 minutes. Chicken should be brown and cooked through; when ready, remove from skillet and slice into thin strips. Cook linguine according to directions on package. Save ½ cup of the pasta cooking water for later. Cook bacon in olive oil in a large skillet until crispy; remove from skillet and discard all but 3 Tbsp. bacon fat. Add onions to skillet and cook over medium-high heat, stirring occasionally, until softened. Add reserved cooking water from pasta to skillet and bring to a boil; stir in linguine and remove from heat. Stir in egg yolks one at a time; add chicken and bacon. Season with pepper and sprinkle with Parmesan.

2. For broccoli: Preheat oven to 450° F. Toss broccoli with olive oil and garlic. Season with salt and pepper, to taste. Spread broccoli evenly on a baking sheet; roast in oven until tender and lightly browned (about 12 minutes). Remove from oven and toss with Parmesan.

3. Serve linguine with a side of broccoli.

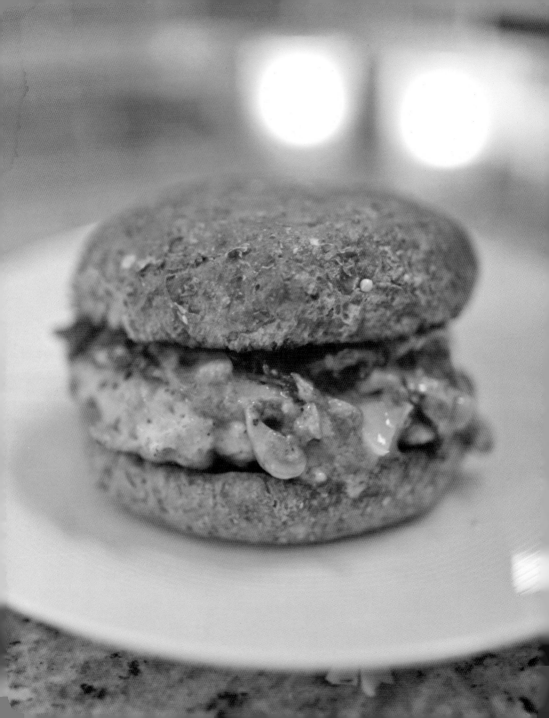

GARLIC-SPINACH TURKEY BURGER

SERVES 4

Antioxidants: garlic, onion, spinach, lemon juice, black pepper, sesame seeds, extra-virgin olive oil, mushrooms

S/C Value = 1/2

 lb. ground turkey

 oz. white mushrooms

 garlic clove, minced

 Tbsp. cornstarch

⁄4 cup unsweetened almond milk

 Tbsp. onion, minced

 cups baby spinach

 tsp. lemon juice

 Tbsp. Parmesan cheese

Salt and pepper, to taste

 Tbsp. extra-virgin olive oil

 Ezekiel 4:9 Sprouted Grain Sesame Burger Buns

. Place ground turkey in a large bowl; season with salt and pepper, to taste. Form into 4 equal-ized patties and transfer to a plate. Cover with plastic wrap and refrigerate for 30 minutes, to llow flavors to blend. Heat mushrooms and garlic in olive oil in a skillet over medium heat for 3–5 minutes. Add in onions and continue to heat, stirring continuously. In a small bowl, mix cornstarch nd almond milk and stir until combined. Add this mixture to the skillet and lower heat. Gradually ncrease heat to medium over time to thicken mixture, and continue to stir. Add in spinach and stir until spinach is wilted. Remove sauce from heat, and add Parmesan cheese and lemon juice; stir until ombined. Remove patties from refrigerator; cook in a skillet over medium heat for 3–5 minutes on ach side, or until lightly browned (turkey should be completely cooked through). Toast rolls.

. Serve patties on rolls topped with sauce with any extra sauce on the side for dipping.

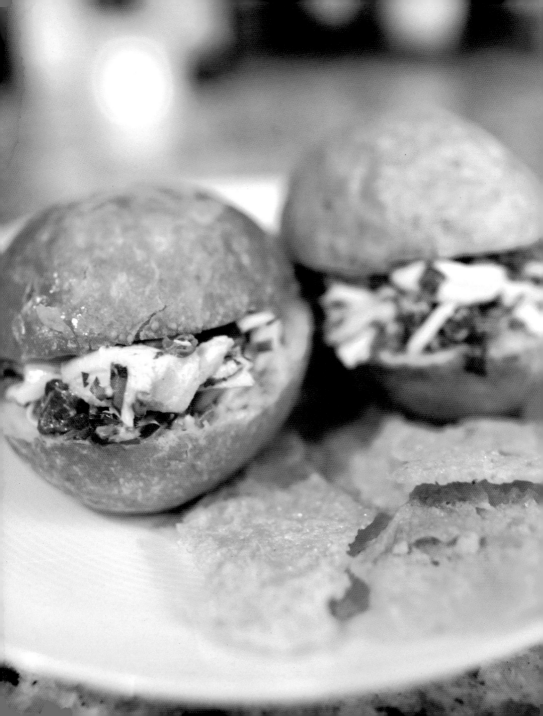

CREAMY CRAB SLIDERS

SERVES 4

Antioxidants: parsley, chives, tarragon, lemon juice, black pepper

S/C Value = 4/2

Sliders:

7 oz. canned crab meat, chopped

¼ cup celery, diced

5 Tbsp. mayonnaise

1 Tbsp. lemon juice

¼ cup Italian parsley, chopped

¼ cup chives, minced

Pinch of fresh tarragon leaves, minced

8 slices American cheese

8 whole-wheat slider rolls

Salt and pepper, to taste

Parmesan crisps:

½ cup Parmesan cheese

1. For sliders: Mix crab, celery, mayo, lemon juice, parsley, chives, and tarragon in a large bowl. Season with salt and pepper, to taste. Chill 1 hour, then remove from refrigerator. Hollow out rolls; toast rolls, then portion crab mixture onto them. Top with cheese, and place under broiler for 3 minutes.

2. For crisps: Heat an 8" pan over medium-low heat. Sprinkle cheese in an even layer, covering the bottom of the pan. Cook 2–3 minutes or until melted; flip and cook 1 minute more. Remove cheese round from pan and place on a cutting board. While still warm, cut round in half with a sharp knife or pizza cutter. Cut each half into 6 wedges, for a total of 12 crisps per round.

3. Serve each person 2 sliders with a side of Parmesan crisps.

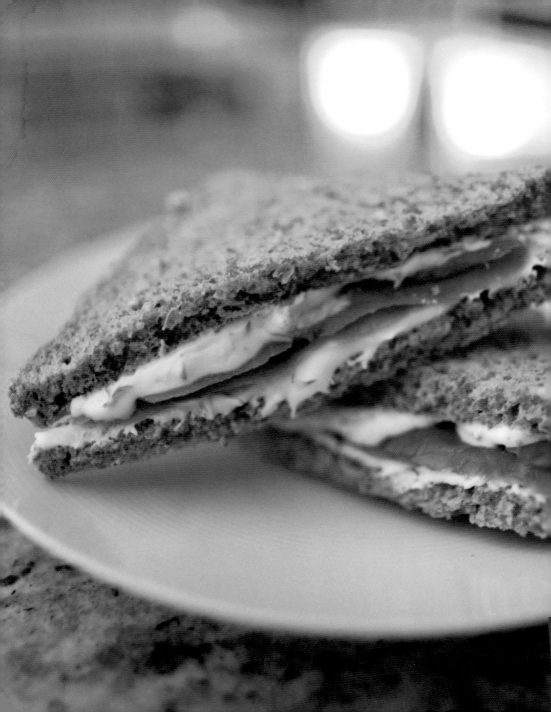

CRÈME FRAÎCHE AND SALMON SANDWICH

SERVES 4

Antioxidant: dill

S/C Value = 1/2

8 slices Food for Life Ezekiel 4:9 Sprouted 100% Whole Grain Bread, toasted
1 cup crème fraîche
1 Tbsp. fresh dill, chopped
16 oz. smoked salmon
Salt, to taste

1. In a small bowl, mix crème fraîche and dill; season with salt, to taste. Spread crème fraîche mixture onto 4 slices of bread and top with salmon. Close sandwiches with remaining bread slices.

2. Cut each sandwich in half before serving.

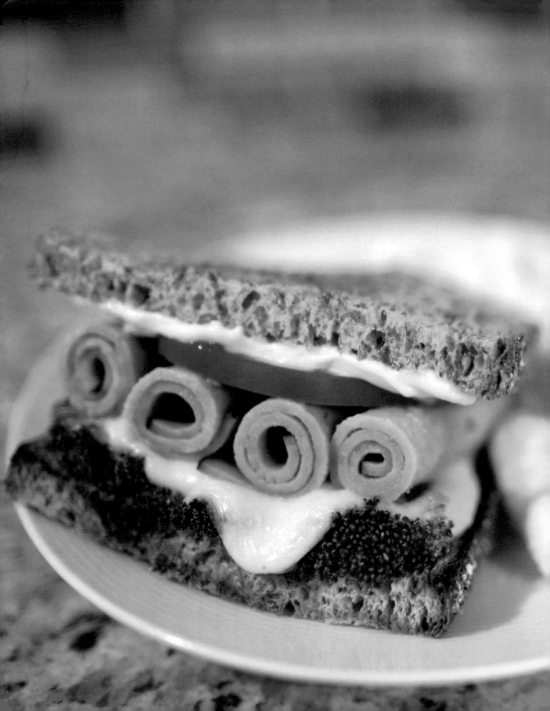

JUICY HAM AND TOMATO SANDWICH

SERVES 4

Antioxidants: broccoli, tomato

S/C Value = 1/2

4 slices Food for Ezekiel 4:9 Sprouted 100% Whole Grain bread, toasted

8 oz. fresh mozzarella, sliced into 1"-thick pieces

4 slices tomato

4 slices ham, deli style

1 cup broccoli florets, chopped

2 oz. Pirate's Booty popcorn

1. Place 1 slice mozzarella on each slice of bread; top with tomato, ham, and broccoli. Place loaded pieces of toast under broiler for 3 minutes. Put 2 toasts on the other 2 pieces of toast to close sandwiches.

2. Cut each sandwich into two halves, and serve each half with a side of Pirate's Booty.

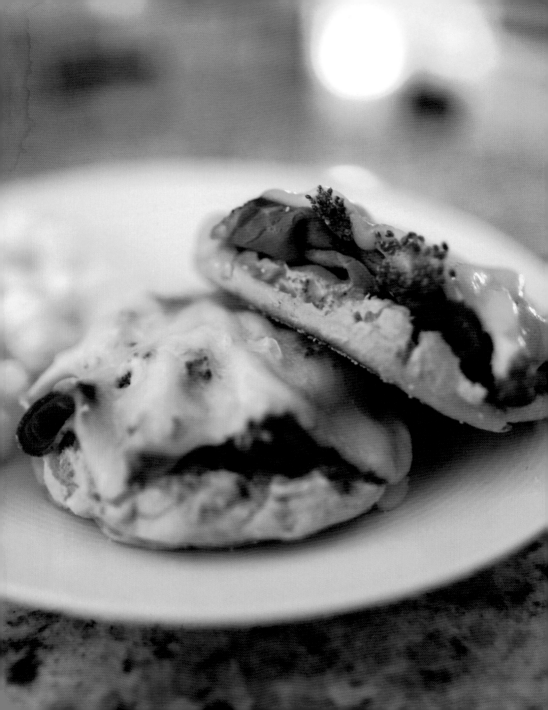

SAVORY ROAST BEEF AND SWISS MELT

SERVES 4

Antioxidant: broccoli

S/C Value = 3/2

4 Rudi's Organic Bakery Whole Grain Wheat English Muffins, halves separated
½ cup mustard
8 slices roast beef
8 slices Swiss cheese, deli style
½ cup broccoli, chopped
2 oz. Pirate's Booty popcorn

1. Spread each English muffin half with 1 Tbsp. mustard. Place roast beef and broccoli on each muffin half, and top with 1 slice of Swiss cheese. Place under broiler for 3 minutes.

2. Serve 2 muffin halves per person with a side of Pirate's Booty.

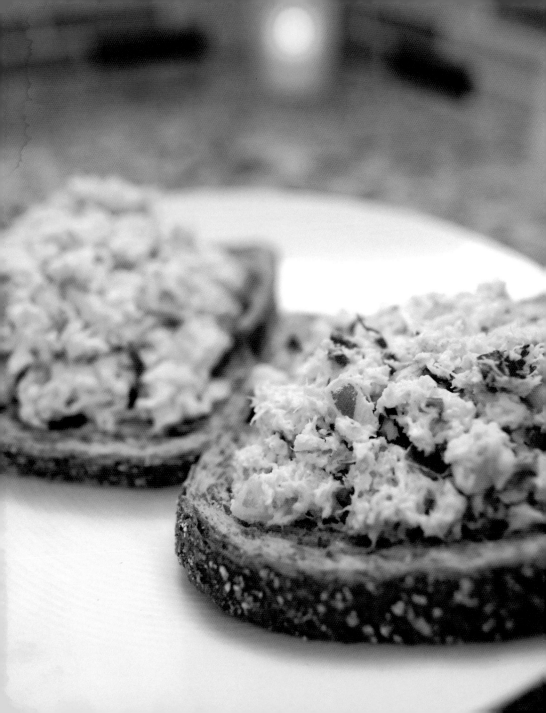

CRISPY CRAB CURRY

SERVES 4

Antioxidants: curry powder, scallions, lime juice

S/C Value = 3/2

8 oz. canned crab meat, chopped
2 Tbsp. mayonnaise
1 Tbsp. lime juice
1 tsp. curry powder
2 scallions, chopped
4 slices Food for Ezekiel 4:9 Sprouted 100% Whole Grain bread, toasted

1. Mix crab meat, mayonnaise, lime juice, curry powder, and scallions in a large salad bowl. Season with salt and pepper, to taste.

2. Serve crab mixture on slices of toasted bread.

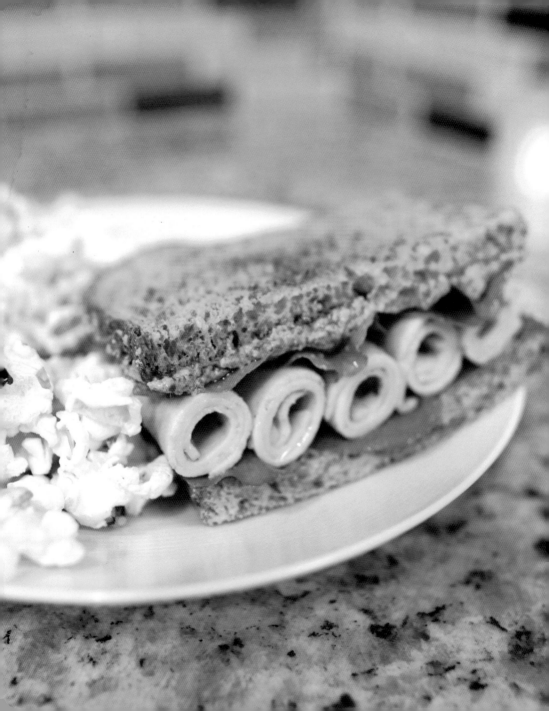

ZESTY PESTO TURKEY WITH PARMESAN POPCORN

SERVES 4

Antioxidants: spinach, basil

S/C Value = 1/2

Sandwich:

8 slices turkey deli meat

¼ cup pesto

¼ cup ricotta cheese

1 cup spinach

4 slices Food for Ezekiel 4:9 Sprouted 100% Whole Grain bread, toasted

Parmesan popcorn:

1 bag microwaveable popcorn

½ cup Parmesan cheese, grated

¼ cup fresh basil, chopped

1. For sandwich: Mix pesto and ricotta in a small bowl. Cut each slice of bread in half; spread pesto and ricotta onto half of slices, top with spinach and turkey, and close with other half-slices of bread.

2. For popcorn: Microwave a bag of popcorn. While it's still hot, add Parmesan and basil, and toss to coat.

3. Serve each half sandwich with a side of popcorn.

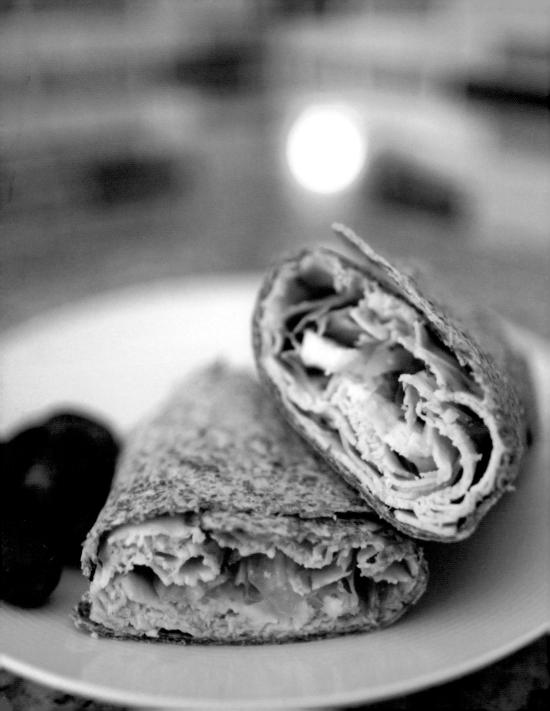

CREAMY CAESAR TURKEY WRAP

SERVES 4

Antioxidants: romaine, red grapes, red bell pepper

S/C Value = 5/1

2 cups romaine lettuce

/4 cup Newman's Own Creamy Caesar Dressing

12 slices turkey, deli style

4 oz. fresh mozzarella cheese, sliced

4 La Tortilla Factory Organic Wheat Tortillas, Low Fat, Carb Cutting

24 red grapes

1. Toss romaine in Caesar dressing in a small bowl. Lay out wraps flat; place mozzarella and turkey on lower half. Top with romaine tossed in Caesar, and fold side flaps toward each other. Roll from the bottom up.

2. Slice each wrap diagonally before serving with equal amounts of grapes.

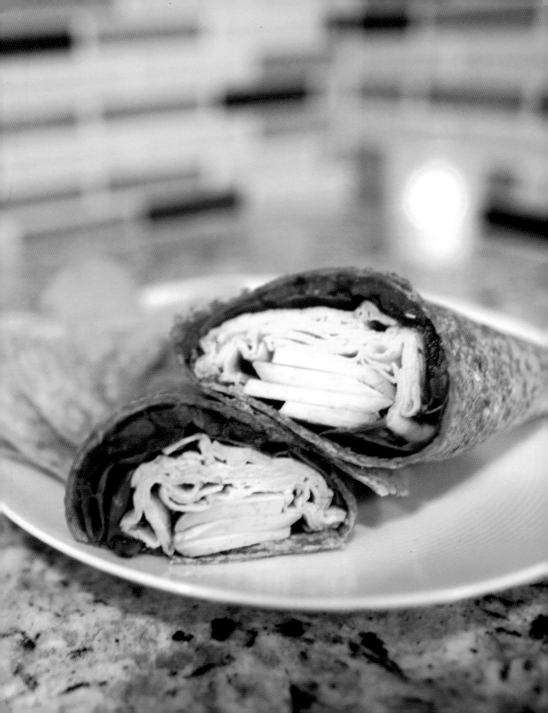

TURKEY AND SALSA WRAP

SERVES 4

Antioxidants: spinach, avocado, salsa

S/C Value = 2/2

4 La Tortilla Factory Organic Wheat Tortillas, Low Fat, Carb Cutting

1 cup salsa

1 cup spinach

12 slices turkey, deli style

1 avocado, sliced

20 Mission Restaurant Style Tortilla Triangles

1. Lay out wraps flat; spread salsa onto each. Place spinach and turkey on lower half of wrap; top with avocado, and fold side flaps toward each other. Roll from the bottom up.

2. Slice each wrap diagonally before serving with tortilla chips.

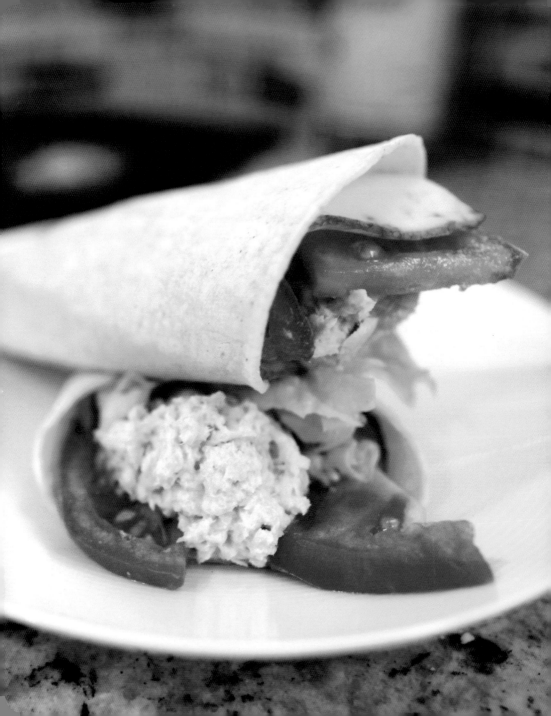

CREAMY TUNA WRAP

SERVES 4

Antioxidants: tuna, tomatoes, lettuce

S/C Value = 3/1

12 oz. canned tuna
/4 cup mayonnaise
2 cups lettuce, shredded
2 medium tomatoes, sliced
4 slices Muenster cheese
4 (6") Mission Yellow or White Corn Tortillas

1. Combine tuna and mayo in a bowl. Lay out wraps flat; place lettuce, tomatoes, and cheese on lower half. Top with tuna, and fold side flaps toward each other. Roll from the bottom up.

2. Slice each wrap diagonally before serving.

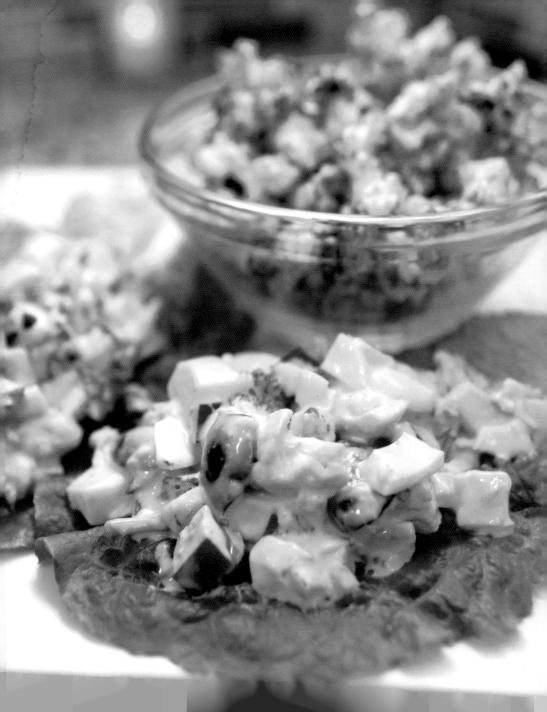

CREAMY EGG-SALAD WRAPS WITH SPICY POPCORN

SERVES 4

Antioxidants: olives, red onion, parsley, capers, black pepper, romaine, turmeric, chili powder

S/C Value = 2/1

Egg-salad wraps:

8 hard-boiled eggs, chopped

¼ cup mayonnaise

8 kalamata olives, chopped

¼ cup red onion, chopped

¼ cup red bell pepper, chopped

2 Tbsp. fresh parsley, chopped

2 Tbsp. drained capers

2 tsp. mustard

Salt and pepper, to taste

4 romaine leaves, torn, for serving

Spicy popcorn:

1 bag microwaveable popcorn

1 Tbsp. butter

1 tsp. turmeric

1 tsp. chili powder

1. For egg salad: Mix eggs, mayo, olives, red onion, bell pepper, parsley, capers, and mustard in a large salad bowl; season with salt and pepper, to taste.

2. For popcorn: Microwave a bag of popcorn. While it's still hot, add butter, turmeric, and chili powder; toss to coat.

3. Serve salad on romaine leaves with a side of popcorn.

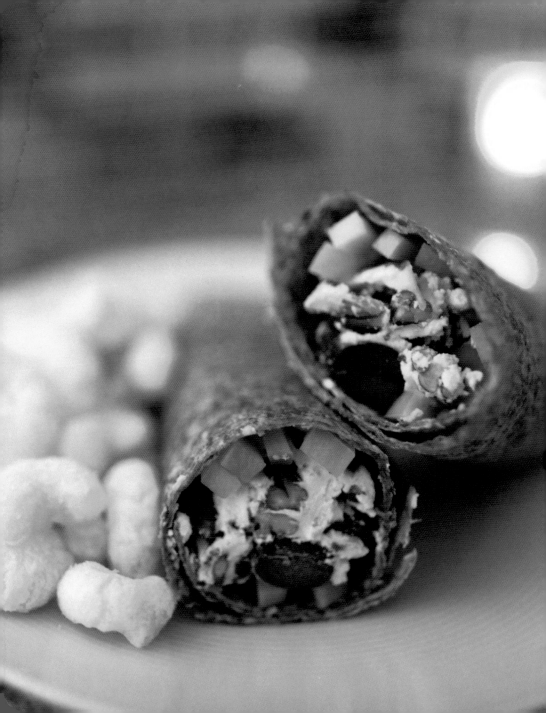

APPLE AND OLIVE WRAP

SERVES 4

Antioxidants: pecans, olives, apple

S/C Value = 4/2

1 cup goat cheese, crumbled
1 cup pecans, chopped
½ apple, sliced very thin
½ cup kalamata olives, sliced in half
4 La Tortilla Factory Organic Wheat Tortillas, Low Fat, Carb Cutting
2 oz. Pirate's Booty popcorn

1. Combine goat cheese, pecans, and olives in a bowl, mashing together with a fork. Lay out wraps flat; place goat-cheese mixture on lower half. Top with apple slices and fold side flaps toward each other. Roll from the bottom up.

2. Slice each wrap diagonally before serving with equal amounts of Pirate's Booty.

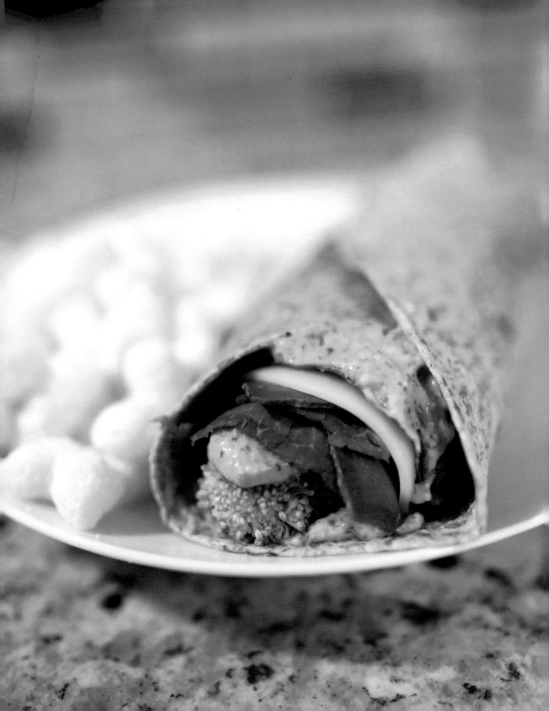

TANGY ROAST-BEEF WRAP

SERVES 4

Antioxidants: broccoli, horseradish

S/C Value = 4/2

2 cups broccoli florets, chopped
¼ cup Annie's Naturals Organic Horseradish Mustard
12 slices roast beef
4 slices provolone cheese, deli style
4 La Tortilla Factory Organic Wheat Tortillas, Low Fat, Carb Cutting
2 oz. Pirate's Booty popcorn

1. Toss broccoli in horseradish mustard in a small bowl. Lay out wraps flat; place provolone and roast beef on lower half. Top with broccoli, and fold side flaps toward each other. Roll from the bottom up.

2. Slice each wrap diagonally before serving with equal amounts of Pirate's Booty.

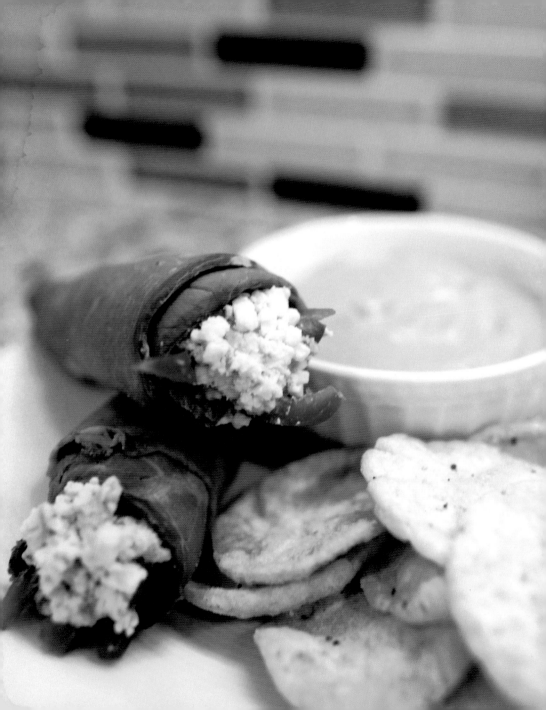

ROBUST ROAST-BEEF WRAPS

SERVES 4

Antioxidants: cayenne pepper, red bell pepper

S/C Value = 1/1

1 cup crumbled blue cheese
Pinch of cayenne pepper
4 slices red bell pepper
4 slices roast beef
2 oz. Salt & Pepper Popchips
Dijon mustard, for serving

1. Place blue cheese in a small bowl and mix with cayenne pepper.
Lay pieces of roast beef out flat; fill each piece with blue cheese and slice of
red bell pepper, and roll. Cut each roll into 2.

2. Serve with each wrap with a side of Popchips and Dijon mustard, for dipping.

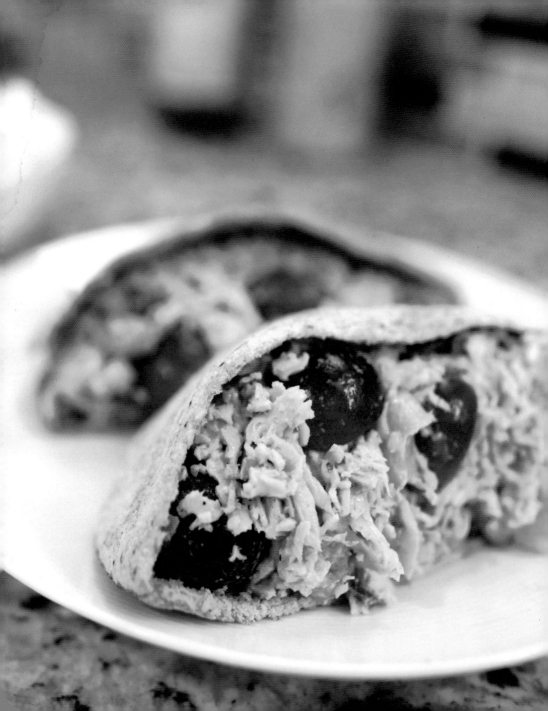

SWEET CURRY TURKEY PITA

SERVES 4

Antioxidants: curry powder, red grapes, scallions, black pepper

S/C Value = 5/2

½ cup mayonnaise

2 tsp. curry powder

4 cups roasted turkey, shredded

½ cup red grapes, halved

4 celery stalks, chopped

2 scallions, chopped

4 (6") Sara Lee Mr. Pita Whole Wheat Pita Breads

Salt and pepper, to taste

1. In a bowl, combine mayo and curry powder; season with salt and pepper, to taste. Add turkey, grapes, celery, and scallion to bowl; mix well. Divide mixture into 4 portions.

2. Slice open pitas, fill with mixture, and serve.

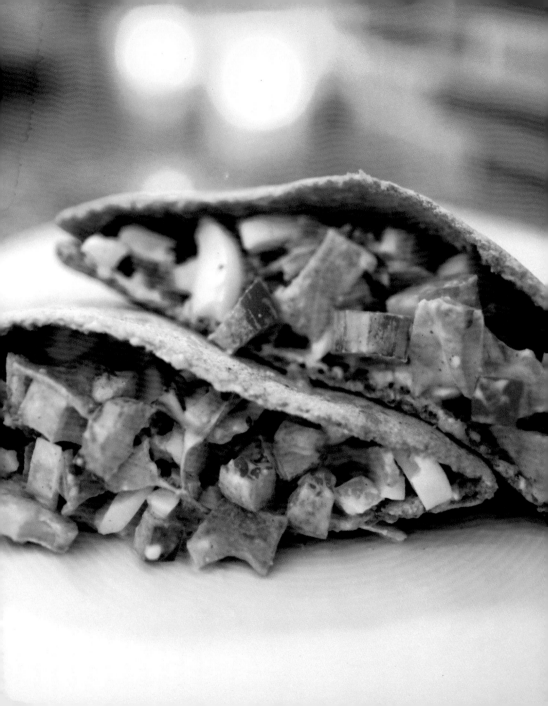

SWEET AND TANGY HAM-SALAD PITA

SERVES 4

Antioxidants: onion, parsley, lemon juice, cayenne pepper, black pepper, red bell pepper

S/C Value = 4/2

8 slices ham, deli style, chopped

4 hard-boiled eggs, chopped

¼ cup pickle, chopped

¼ cup mayonnaise

2 Tbsp. onion, minced

2 Tbsp. celery, minced

2 Tbsp. red bell pepper, minced

1 Tbsp. fresh parsley, chopped

2 tsp. Dijon mustard

1 Tbsp. lemon juice

Cayenne pepper, to taste

Salt and pepper, to taste

4 (6") Sara Lee Mr. Pita Whole Wheat Pita Breads

1. Mix all ingredients but pitas, cayenne pepper, salt, and pepper together in a large salad bowl. Season with cayenne pepper, salt, and pepper, to taste.

2. Slice open pitas, fill with mixture, and serve.

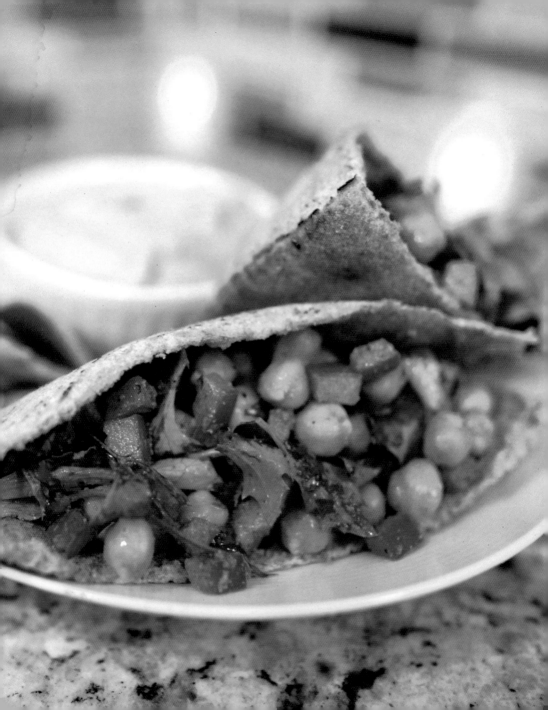

SAVORY CURRY CHICKPEA PITA

SERVES 4

Antioxidants: curry powder, cumin, extra-virgin olive oil, cilantro, lime juice, red bell pepper, mixed greens, chickpeas

S/C Value = 2/2

1 tsp. Bragg's apple cider vinegar

1 Tbsp. lime juice

1 tsp. curry powder

1 tsp. cumin

2 Tbsp. extra-virgin olive oil

1 can chickpeas (about 8 oz.), rinsed and drained

½ red bell pepper, chopped

¼ cup fresh cilantro, chopped

1 cup mixed greens

Salt, to taste

4 (6") Sara Lee Mr. Pita Whole Wheat Pita Breads

20 Stacy's Simply Naked Pita Chips

4 Tbsp. Sabra hummus

1. Mix apple cider vinegar, lime juice, curry powder, cumin, and olive oil in a large salad bowl. Add chickpeas, bell pepper, cilantro, and mixed greens; toss to combine. Season with salt, to taste.

2. Slice open pitas, fill with mixture, and serve each with 5 chips and 1 Tbsp. hummus on the side.

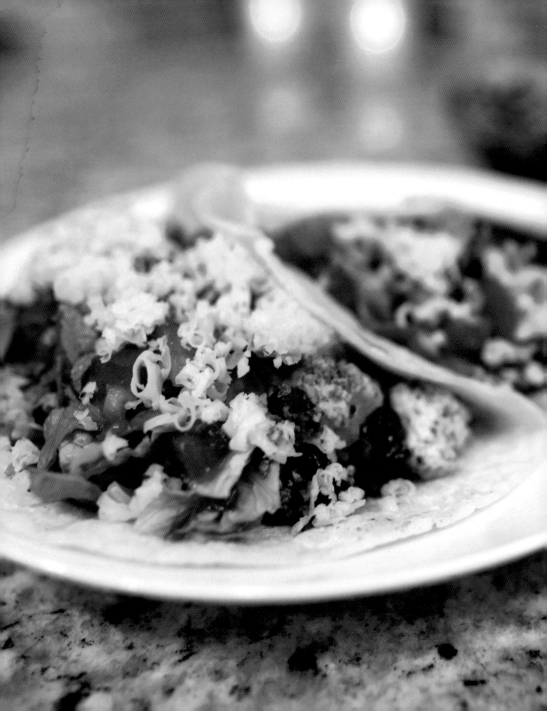

SPICY TOFU TACOS

SERVES 4

Antioxidants: chili powder, oregano, cumin, coriander, garlic, scallions, extra-virgin olive oil, romaine, tomatoes, black beans

S/C Value = 2/2

10 oz. extra-firm tofu, drained
1 tsp. chili powder
½ tsp. oregano
½ tsp. ground cumin
½ tsp. ground coriander
Salt, to taste
2 garlic cloves, chopped
2 scallions, chopped
1 Tbsp. extra-virgin olive oil
10 oz. black beans, drained and rinsed
8 (6") Mission Yellow Corn Tortillas
2 cups romaine lettuce, shredded
1 cup tomatoes, chopped
1 cup cheddar cheese, shredded

1. Mash tofu, chili powder, oregano, cumin, and coriander in a bowl with a fork. Season with salt, to taste, and set aside. Cook garlic and 1 scallion in olive oil in a skillet over medium heat for 2–3 minutes. Add tofu mixture; cook until most of the moisture has evaporated (about 10–12 minutes), stirring occasionally. Add beans and remaining scallion and stir. Cook until beans are heated throughout, about 3 minutes.

2. Spoon tofu mixture into tortillas; top with lettuce, tomatoes, and cheese. Serve.

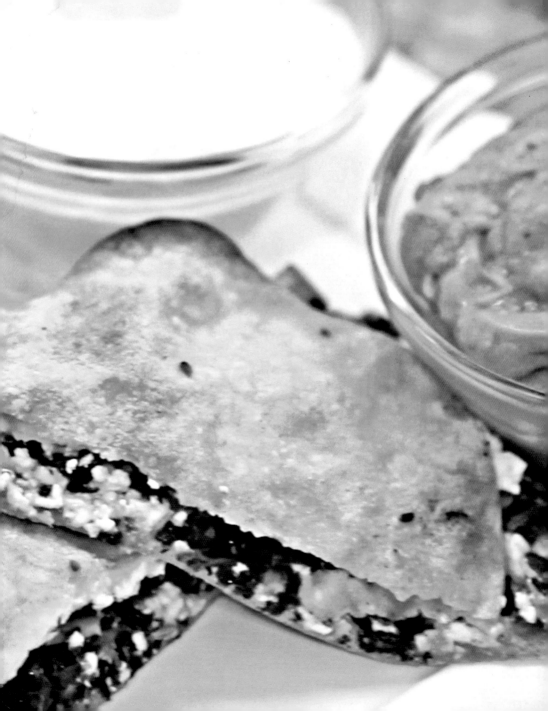

SIZZLING SPINACH-MUSHROOM QUESADILLA

SERVES 4

Antioxidants: spinach, cumin, coriander, extra-virgin olive oil, salsa, guacamole

S/C Value = 3/2

6 oz. mushrooms, sliced

1 Tbsp. extra-virgin olive oil (plus extra, as needed)

8 oz. frozen chopped spinach, drained and squeezed dry

½ fresh jalapeño pepper, chopped

½ tsp. ground cumin

¼ tsp. ground coriander

Salt, to taste

8 (6") Mission Yellow Corn Tortillas

6 oz. feta cheese

Salsa, for serving

Sour cream, for serving

Guacamole, for serving

1. Preheat oven to 450° F. Cook mushrooms in olive oil in a skillet over medium-high heat until browned (about 7 minutes). Add spinach, jalapeño, cumin, and coriander to skillet; season with salt, to taste. Brush tortillas with olive oil; lay 4 on baking sheet. Top tortillas evenly with mushroom-spinach-jalapeño mixture; add feta. Cover with remaining tortillas, pressing down firmly. Bake until tortillas begin to crisp, about 12 minutes.

2. Cut each into wedges and serve with salsa, sour cream, and guacamole.

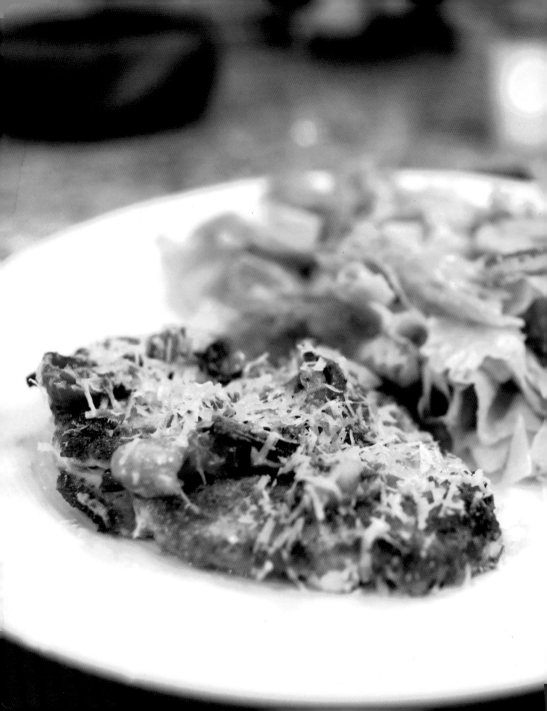

CRISPY CHICKEN PARMESAN

SERVES 4

Antioxidants: tomatoes, basil, shallots, extra-virgin olive oil, black pepper, romaine

S/C Value = 2/2

Chicken:

4 skinless, boneless chicken-breast
   cutlets

½ cup cherry tomatoes, halved

½ cup fresh basil, chopped

½ cup shallots, sliced

½ cup whole-wheat bread crumbs

¼ cup Parmesan cheese, grated

2 Tbsp. extra-virgin olive oil

Salt and pepper, to taste

Salad:

2 cups romaine lettuce

1 cup Parmesan cheese, grated

1 cup croutons

¼ cup Newman's Own Creamy
   Caesar Dressing

Salt and pepper, to taste

1. For chicken: Place cutlets on a flat surface and lay a sheet of plastic wrap over them; pound flat with a mallet. Cook tomatoes, basil, and shallots in 1 Tbsp. olive oil in a skillet over medium heat for 10 minutes. Season with salt and pepper, to taste, and stir; remove from heat and set aside. Mix bread crumbs and 2 Tbsp. of Parmesan cheese in a bowl; season with salt and pepper, to taste. Cover each chicken breast with this mixture. Cook chicken in remaining olive oil in a second skillet, over medium heat for 5–8 minutes (it should be brown and cooked through). Remove chicken from heat; spoon tomato mixture over each piece. Top with Parmesan cheese, allowing the cheese to melt for several minutes before serving.

2. For salad: Mix romaine, Parmesan, and croutons in a large salad bowl. Season with salt and pepper, to taste. Toss with Caesar dressing.

3. Serve each chicken breast with a side of salad.

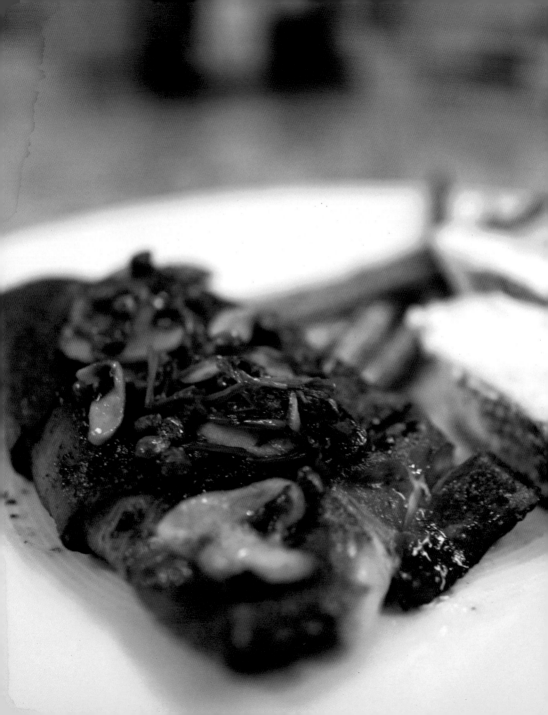

SAVORY SAGE CHICKEN MARSALA

SERVES 4

Antioxidants: sage, wine, capers, parsley, extra-virgin olive oil, black pepper, mushrooms

S/C Value = 4/2

12 fresh sage leaves

12 slices prosciutto

4 chicken breasts

2 Tbsp. whole-wheat flour

2 Tbsp. extra-virgin olive oil

3 Tbsp. butter

1 cup mushrooms, sliced

¾ cup marsala wine

2 Tbsp. capers in brine, chopped

2 Tbsp. parsley, chopped

Salt and pepper, to taste

8" baguette, cut into 4 portions

1. Preheat oven to 350° F. Place a sage leaf in the center of each slice of prosciutto; wrap each chicken breast with 3 of these slices. Sprinkle flour and pepper onto breasts. Cook chicken in 1 Tbsp. olive oil and 2 Tbsp. butter in a skillet over medium heat, for about 3 minutes each side (chicken should be golden brown). Transfer to a baking sheet. Cook mushrooms in remaining olive oil in a separate skillet over medium heat until tender; remove mushrooms and set aside. Transfer baking sheet to oven; cook chicken for 5 minutes. While chicken is cooking, take the skillet the chicken was cooked in and turn heat to medium-low. Add marsala and simmer for 3 minutes, stirring consistently. Some bits will brown; scrape and continue to stir. Add capers and parsley; stir in remaining tablespoon of butter and add mushrooms. Remove chicken from oven.

2. Spoon sauce over chicken and serve with a small piece of baguette.

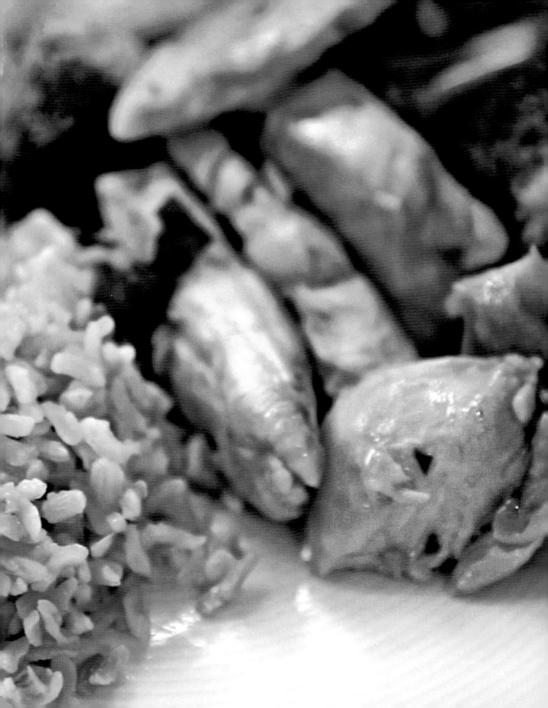

CHICKEN AND BROCCOLI STIR-FRY

SERVES 4

Antioxidants: garlic, ginger, broccoli, extra-virgin olive oil

S/C Value = 2/2

¾ cup chicken broth

3 Tbsp. soy sauce

1 tsp. rice vinegar

¼ tsp. red pepper flakes

2 tsp. cornstarch

1 lb. boneless, skinless chicken tenderloins, cut into strips

2 Tbsp. extra-virgin olive oil

4 garlic cloves, minced

3 Tbsp. peeled fresh ginger, minced

3 cups broccoli florets

2 cups (as prepared) rice

1. Mix broth, soy sauce, vinegar, red pepper flakes, and cornstarch in a bowl. Heat chicken in 1 Tbsp. olive oil in a wok on high heat; stir-fry until somewhat browned (about 3 minutes). Remove from wok and set aside. Add garlic and ginger to the wok with the remaining olive oil; stir-fry for 30 seconds. Add broccoli and stir-fry for 3 minutes. Finally, add soy mixture and chicken; stir well and cover. Lower heat to medium and simmer until broccoli is tender (about 3 minutes). Prepare rice according to directions on packaging.

2. Serve each portion of chicken and broccoli with a side of rice.

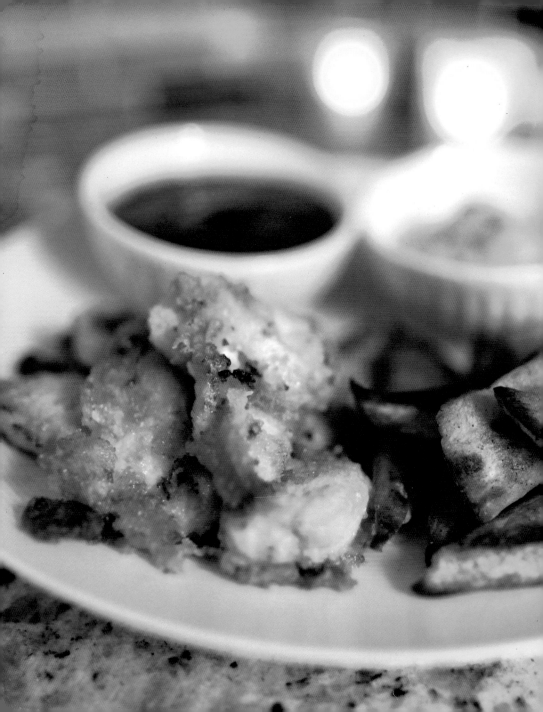

CRISPY CHICKEN STRIPS

SERVES 4

Antioxidants: extra-virgin olive oil, black pepper, cayenne pepper, sweet potatoes

S/C Value = 4/2

Chicken strips:

2 chicken breasts, cut into bite-sized pieces

6 Tbsp. whole-wheat bread crumbs

2 Tbsp. panko

2 Tbsp. Parmesan cheese, grated

Extra-virgin olive oil, as needed

Salt and pepper, to taste

Nature's Hollow sugar-free ketchup, for serving

Dijon mustard, for serving

Sweet-potato fries:

2 sweet potatoes, peeled and cut into fry-size wedges

Pinch of cayenne pepper

½ tsp. paprika

1 Tbsp. extra-virgin olive oil

Salt and pepper, to taste

1. For chicken: Preheat oven to 425° F. Lightly oil a baking sheet. Mix bread crumbs, panko, and Parmesan in a bowl. Drizzle chicken pieces in olive oil and season with salt and pepper, to taste. Coat each piece of chicken in bread-crumb mixture by dipping into bowl. Place pieces of chicken on baking sheet; bake 8–10 minutes. Turn pieces over and cook an additional 3–5 minutes, or until cooked through.

2. For fries: Mix cayenne pepper, paprika, olive oil, salt, and pepper in a small dish. Coat each sweet-potato wedge in this mixture by tossing in bowl; place wedges on a baking sheet. Bake at 425° F for 25 minutes, turning halfway through, or until sweet potatoes have browned on the outside.

3. Serve chicken strips with a side of fries and ketchup and mustard for dipping.

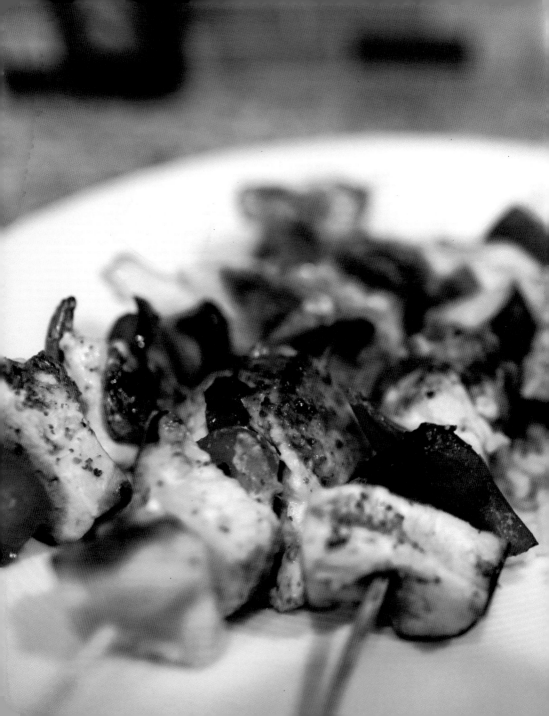

SPICY CHICKEN KEBABS

SERVES 4

Antioxidants: lemon juice, scallions, extra-virgin olive oil, black pepper, mushrooms, red bell peppers, eggplant, onion

S/C Value = 4/2

¼ cup horseradish mustard, plus extra for dipping

1½ Tbsp. lemon juice

1½ Tbsp. extra-virgin olive oil

3 chicken breasts, cut into 1½" pieces

½ lb. button mushrooms

½ eggplant, cut into 1½" pieces

½ onion, cut into 1½" pieces

½ red bell pepper, cut into 1½" pieces

Salt and pepper, to taste

2 cups (as prepared) brown rice

1. Soak wooden skewers in water for 20 to 30 minutes. In a small bowl, mix together mustard, lemon juice, and olive oil. Season with salt and pepper, to taste. Slide chicken, mushrooms, eggplant, onions, and peppers onto skewers. Brush chicken and veggies with mustard mixture. Cook skewers in a skillet over medium heat, turning frequently, until chicken is cooked and vegetables are tender (about 10 minutes). Prepare rice according to directions on packaging.

2. Serve skewers with a side of rice and additional horseradish mustard for dipping.

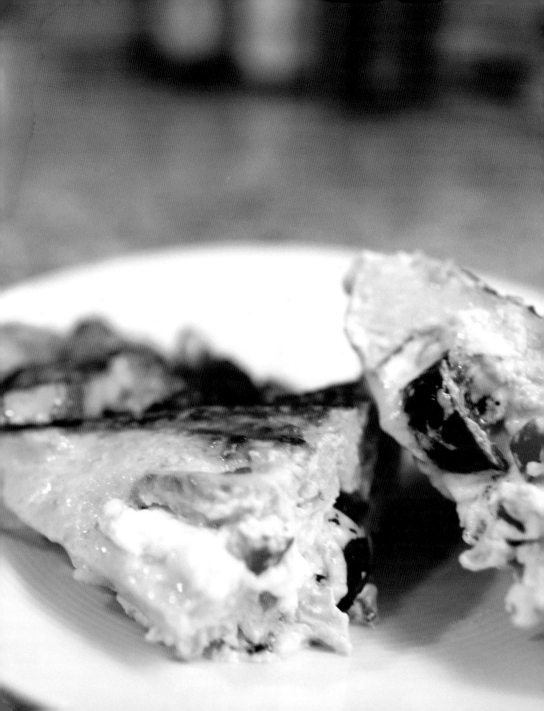

CREAMY GOAT-CHEESE STUFFED CHICKEN

SERVES 4

Antioxidants: thyme, extra-virgin olive oil, black pepper, olives, red bell peppers

S/C Value = 2/1

Chicken:

3 oz. goat cheese

¼ cup olives

1 red pepper, chopped

1 Tbsp. fresh thyme, chopped

4 chicken breasts

2 Tbsp. extra-virgin olive oil
   (plus extra, as needed)

Salt and pepper, to taste

Sautéed zucchini:

1 cup zucchini, sliced

1 Tbsp. extra-virgin olive oil

Salt and pepper, to taste

1. For chicken: Mix goat cheese, olives, red pepper, and thyme together in a small bowl; season with salt and pepper, to taste. Make a slit in each chicken breast and fill with cheese mixture. Brush the breasts with olive oil; season with salt and pepper, to taste. Secure chicken with toothpicks, and cook in 2 Tbsp. olive oil for 5–8 minutes in a skillet over medium heat. (Chicken should be browned and cooked through.)

2. For zucchini: Cook in olive oil in a skillet until tender (about 3–5 minutes). Remove from heat and season with salt and pepper, to taste.

3. Serve each chicken breast with a side of zucchini.

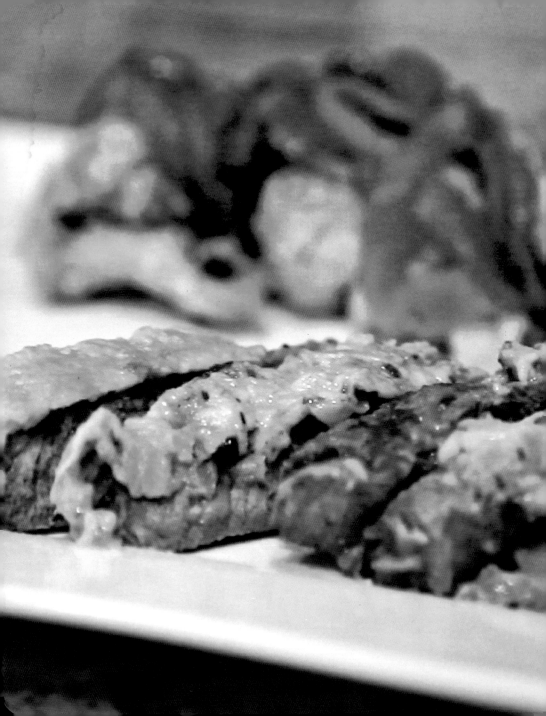

GARLIC-GRILLED RIB EYE

SERVES 4

Antioxidants: garlic, thyme, extra-virgin olive oil, black pepper, cauliflower, capers, parsley, red peppers

S/C Value = 4/1

Steak:

12 garlic cloves

2 Tbsp. fresh thyme leaves, chopped

2 Tbsp. Dijon mustard

2 cups Parmesan cheese, grated

2 rib eye steaks (each about 2–2½" thick)

1 Tbsp. extra-virgin olive oil (plus extra, as needed)

Salt and pepper, to taste

Cauliflower:

1 lb. cauliflower crowns, broken into small florets

2 garlic cloves, minced

½ tsp. crushed red pepper

1 Tbsp. capers, undrained

¼ cup roasted red peppers

¼ cup fresh parsley, chopped

⅛ cup pine nuts

3 Tbsp. extra-virgin olive oil

Salt and pepper, to taste

1. For steak: Preheat oven to 425° F. Cook garlic in olive oil in a skillet over medium heat for 5–10 minutes, or until brown. Remove cloves and let cool before breaking up with fork in a bowl. Add thyme and mash into one mixture. Mix in Dijon mustard; season with salt and pepper, to taste. Drizzle steaks with olive oil and season with salt and pepper, to taste. Cook steaks in a skillet on high heat, about 5 minutes each side; remove from heat and place on a large baking sheet. Cover tops of steaks generously with garlic-and-mustard mixture; top with Parmesan. Place steaks in oven and cook for 8–10 minutes. After removing from oven, let rest a few minutes, then slice each steak in half.

2. For cauliflower: Toss florets with 2 Tbsp. olive oil and season with salt and pepper, to taste. Arrange in a single layer on a baking sheet; bake at 425° for 25 minutes, or until tender. Cook garlic in remaining olive oil in a skillet over medium heat for 1 minute. Add crushed red pepper, capers, and peppers to skillet; cook for an additional minute, stirring constantly. Add in parsley and cauliflower and cook for another minute, stirring constantly. Season with salt and pepper, to taste. Garnish with pine nuts before serving.

3. Serve each half of a steak with a side of cauliflower.

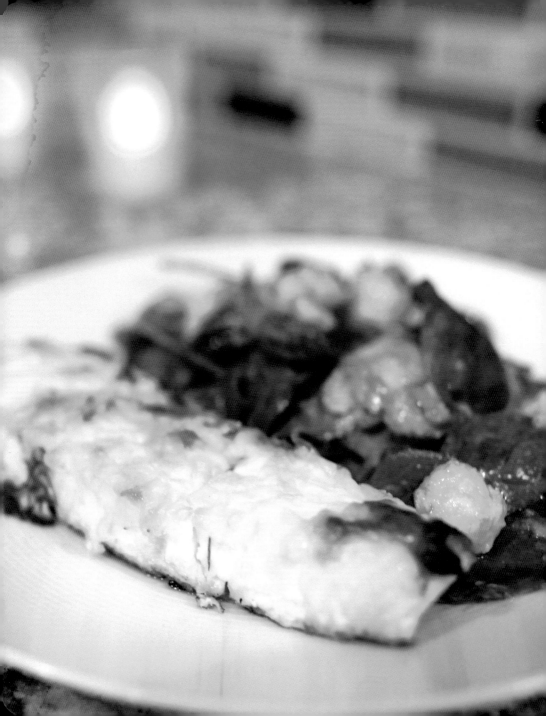

PARMESAN DILL HALIBUT

SERVES 4

Antioxidants: garlic, dill, black pepper, spinach, macadamia nuts, avocado

S/C Value = 3/1

Halibut:

4 halibut fillets

½ cup sour cream

1 garlic clove, minced

½ tsp. dill weed

½ cup Parmesan cheese, grated

Salt and pepper, to taste

Avocado and Macadamia Nut Salad:

2 cups baby spinach

1 cup macadamia nuts

1 avocado, sliced

¼ cup Newman's Own Balsamic Vinaigrette Dressing

1. For halibut: Preheat oven to 375° F. Combine sour cream, garlic, and dill weed in a small bowl; stir in Parmesan, and season with salt and pepper, to taste. Place fish in a baking dish; spread an even coating of the mixture over each piece. Bake fish for 22–24 minutes, or until pieces feel firm but not hard to the touch.

2. For salad: Place spinach in a large salad bowl. Toss with vinaigrette dressing; season with salt and pepper, to taste. Divide onto four plates and top with avocado and macadamia nuts.

3. Serve each piece of fish with a side of salad.

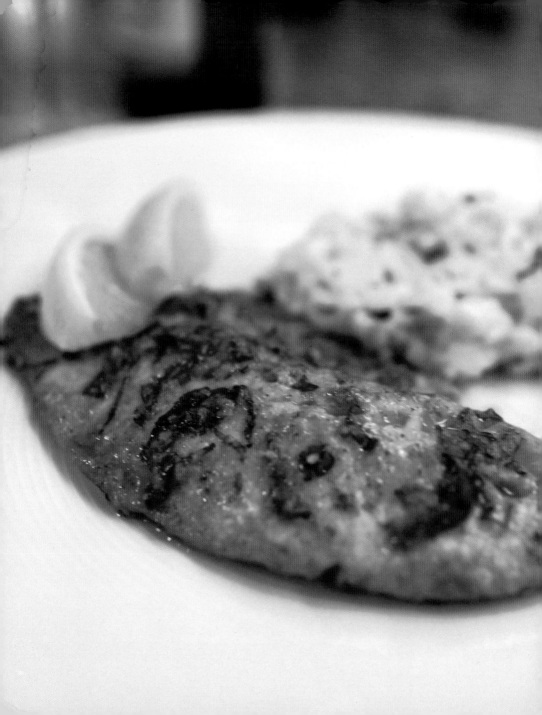

PARMESAN TILAPIA WITH MINT RISOTTO

SERVES 4

Antioxidants: cayenne pepper, parsley, extra-virgin olive oil, black pepper, mint, lemon juice

S/C Value = 1/1

Tilapia:

1 cup Parmesan cheese, grated

1 tsp. cayenne pepper

1 Tbsp. fresh parsley, chopped

4 tilapia fillets

Extra-virgin olive oil, as needed

Salt and pepper, to taste

Mint risotto:

1 cup risotto

1⅓ cups chicken stock

⅔ cup white wine

½ cup sour cream

3 Tbsp. butter

Half a handful mint leaves, chopped

Salt and pepper, to taste

Other sides:

Lemon wedges, for serving

1. For tilapia: Preheat the oven to 400° F. In a bowl, combine Parmesan, cayenne pepper, and parsley; season with salt and pepper, to taste. Drizzle the fish with olive oil and cover in Parmesan mixture. Line a baking sheet with aluminum foil; place fish on it and bake until opaque in the thickest part (about 10–12 minutes).

2. For risotto: Bring half of the stock to a boil; add risotto. Return to a boil, stirring continuously. Turn heat down and simmer until almost all stock has been absorbed. Add rest of stock and the white wine until risotto is cooked. Turn off heat, and add butter and mint leaves; season with salt and pepper, to taste. Put a lid on the pan until ready to serve.

3. Serve fish with a side of risotto and lemon wedges, for garnish.

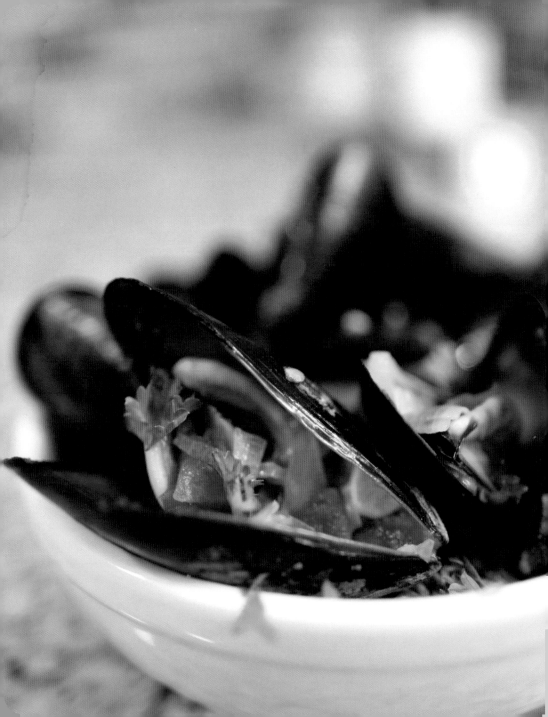

GARLIC AND SAFFRON MUSSELS

SERVES 4

Antioxidants: shallots, garlic, tomatoes, parsley, black pepper

S/C Value = 2/1

3 lbs. fresh mussels

1 large pinch saffron (about 30 threads)

¾ cup dry white wine

2 Tbsp. butter

2 medium shallots, sliced

2 garlic cloves, sliced

2 medium tomatoes, chopped

¼ cup fresh parsley, chopped

Salt and pepper, to taste

1. Holding mussels under cool running water, scrub with a stiff sponge. Debeard by gripping the tough fibers extending from the shell and pull to remove; discard beards. Steep the saffron in the wine for 10 minutes. Meanwhile, melt the butter over medium heat in a shallow stockpot; once it's foamy, add shallots, garlic, and ½ teaspoon salt. Cook until shallots are transparent and garlic is soft (about 3 minutes), stirring every so often to keep the garlic from scorching. Pour in the wine and saffron; add the tomatoes and return to a simmer, stirring once or twice. Add the mussels and cover tightly; cook until they all open (about 6 minutes), stirring once about halfway through. Discard any unopened mussels. Taste the broth, and season with salt and pepper.

2. Spoon the mussels and broth into bowls and sprinkle with parsley before serving.

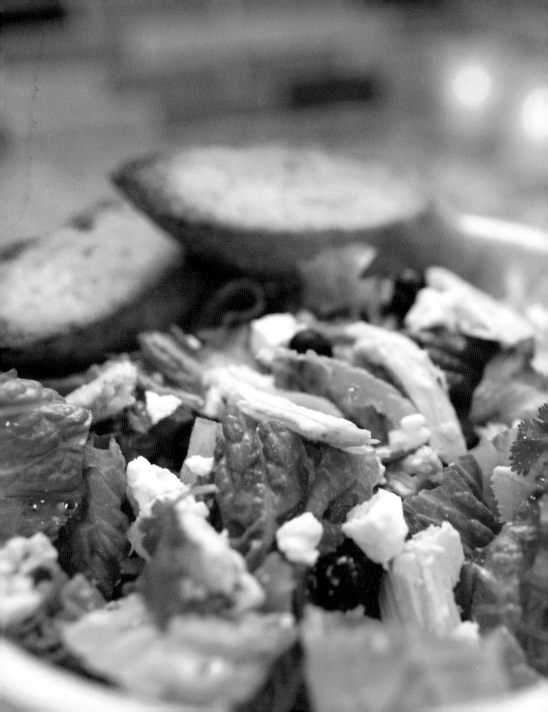

SUMMER BLUEBERRY CHICKEN SALAD

SERVES 4

Antioxidants: blueberries, cilantro, black pepper

S/C Value = 5/1

4 handfuls of meat from a rotisserie chicken
1 cup blueberries
1 cup feta cheese, crumbled
¼ cup cilantro, chopped
4 cups butter lettuce
¼ cup low-sugar Italian dressing
Salt and pepper, to taste

1. Place lettuce in a large bowl and toss with dressing. Divide lettuce onto 4 plates. Mix blueberries, feta, and cilantro in a small bowl; season with salt and pepper, to taste. Top salad with blueberry mixture, then place 1 handful of chicken onto each salad.

2. Serve chilled.

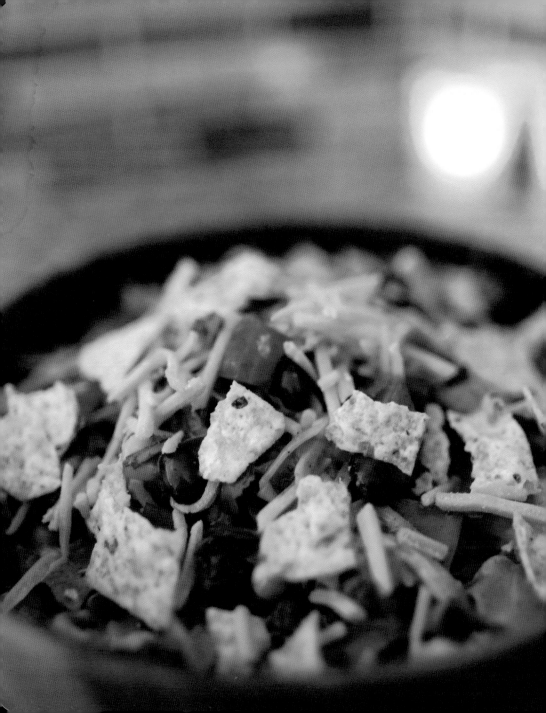

RANCH BBQ CHOPPED SALAD

SERVES 4

Antioxidants: romaine, tomato, cilantro, black beans

S/C Value = 3/2

4 cups romaine lettuce, shredded
1 tomato, chopped
1 cup fresh cilantro, chopped
1 cup canned corn, drained
1 can (15 oz.) black beans, drained
1 cup cheddar cheese, shredded
10 crushed tortilla chips
½ cup Newman's Own Ranch Dressing
¼ cup Scott's BBQ Sauce

1. Mix romaine, tomato, cilantro, corn, black beans, and cheddar cheese in a large salad bowl. In a small bowl, mix ranch dressing and BBQ sauce. Toss salad with ranch-and-BBQ mixture, and divide among 4 plates.

2. Top with crushed tortilla chips before serving.

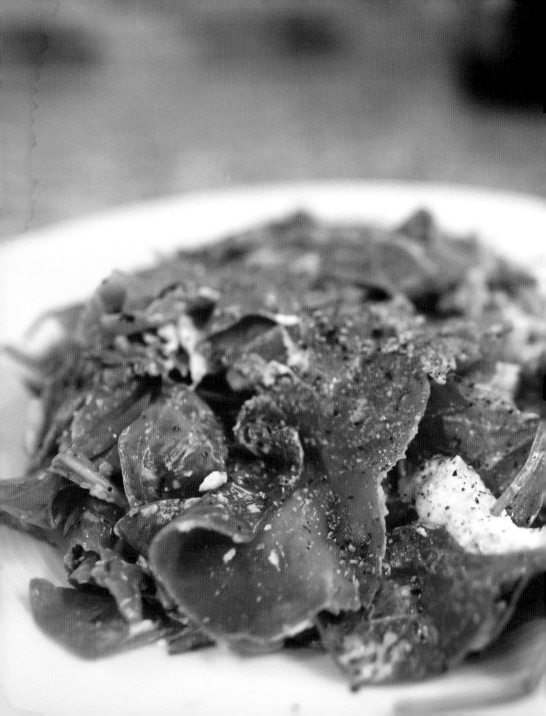

PROSCIUTTO AND GOAT CHEESE SALAD

SERVES 4

Antioxidants: spinach, black pepper

S/C Value = 2/1

8 cups baby spinach
8 slices prosciutto, cut into thin strips
½ cup pine nuts
½ cup crumbled goat cheese
¼ cup Annie's Naturals Organic Balsamic Vinaigrette
4 slices Wasa Multi Grain crispbread
Salt and pepper, to taste

1. Mix spinach, prosciutto, pine nuts, and goat cheese in a large salad bowl; toss with dressing and season with salt and pepper, to taste. Divide among 4 plates.

2. Crumble 1 slice of crispbread over each salad to serve as croutons before serving.

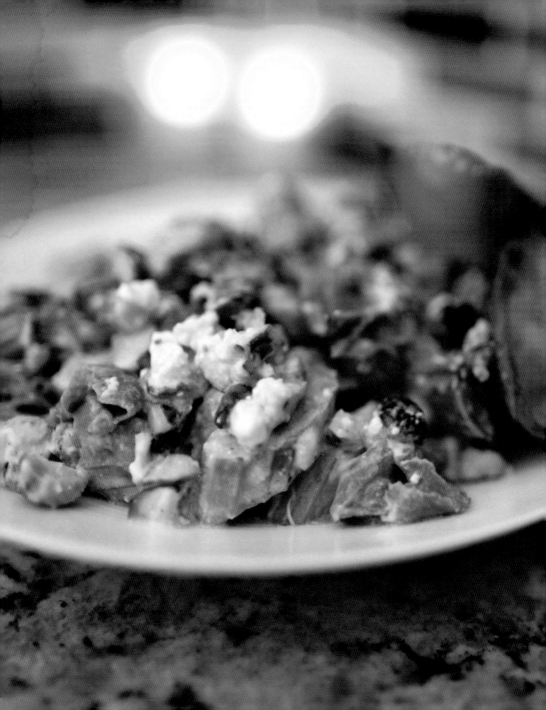

RICH ROAST BEEF AND HAZELNUT SALAD

SERVES 4

Antioxidants: hazelnuts, extra-virgin olive oil, lemon juice, black pepper

S/C Value = 4/2

2 bunches celery stalks

8 slices roast beef, chopped

1 cup hazelnuts, chopped

2 cups blue cheese, crumbled, at room temperature

2 Tbsp. lemon juice

2 Tbsp. extra-virgin olive oil (plus extra, as needed)

Salt and pepper, to taste

8" baguette, cut into 4 portions

1. Remove tops from bunches of celery, and slice stalks on the diagonal into ¼"-thick slices. Mix celery, roast beef, hazelnuts, and blue cheese together in a large salad bowl. In a small bowl, mix lemon juice and olive oil; season with salt and pepper, to taste. Toss salad with lemon-juice-and-olive-oil mixture. Transfer salad to baking dish and place under broiler for 5 minutes to warm, tossing once halfway through. Brush baguette pieces with olive oil and place under broiler for 3 minutes to toast.

2. Serve each salad with 1 slice of baguette.

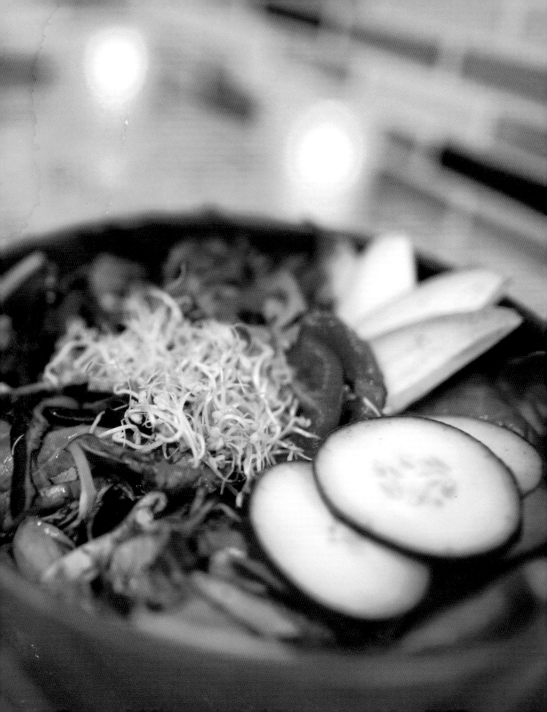

FRESH AND SPICY GARDEN SALAD

SERVES 4

Antioxidants: spinach, avocado, sprouts, cilantro, basil, cayenne pepper, lemon juice, black pepper, red peppers, red cabbage

S/C Value = 3/2

1 cup baby spinach
1 cucumber, sliced
½ cup roasted red peppers
2 avocados
1 cup red cabbage, chopped
¼ cup sprouts (broccoli or other)
1 cup cilantro, chopped
1 cup fresh basil, chopped
½ tsp. cayenne pepper
1 Tbsp. lemon juice
Tabasco sauce, to taste
Salt and pepper, to taste
4 oz. Rold Gold Classic Style Pretzel Thins
   (about 32 pretzels)
Mustard, for dipping

1. Mix spinach, cucumber, roasted red pepper, avocado, red cabbage, sprouts, cilantro, and basil in a large salad bowl. Season with cayenne pepper, salt, and pepper, to taste. In a small bowl, mix lemon juice and Tabasco; toss salad with this mixture.

2. Serve salad with pretzels with mustard, for dipping.

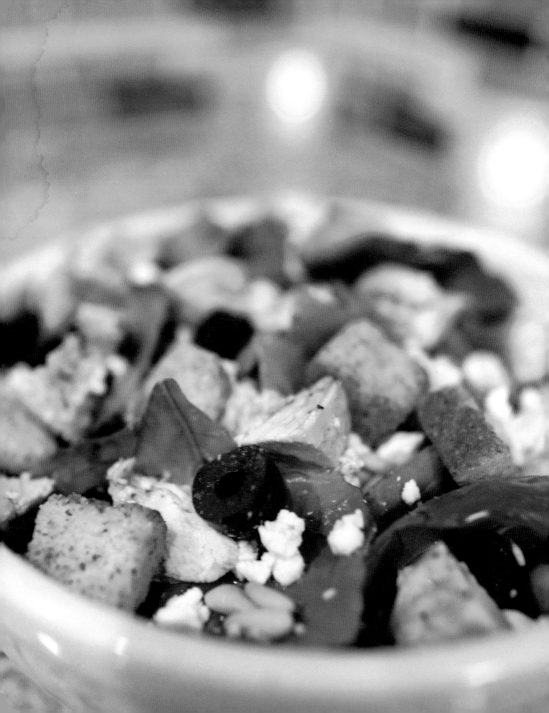

TANGY GREEK ARUGULA SALAD

SERVES 4

Antioxidants: olives, arugula, red wine vinegar, black pepper

S/C Value = 1/1

½ cup pine nuts

1 cup kalamata olives, pitted and halved

1 cup goat cheese, crumbled

4 handfuls of meat from a rotisserie chicken

2 cups arugula

1 cup croutons, plus extra for serving

¼ cup red wine vinegar

Salt and pepper, to taste

1. Mix pine nuts, olives, goat cheese, chicken, and arugula in a large salad bowl; season with salt and pepper, to taste. Toss with red wine vinegar.

2. Top with croutons and serve.

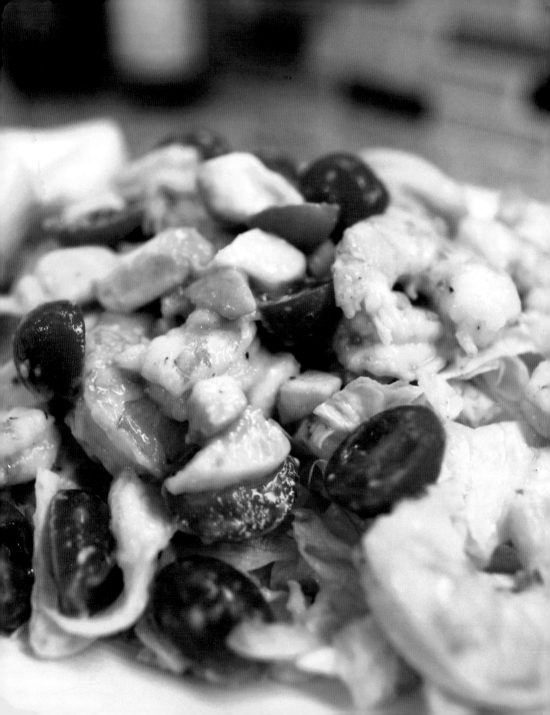

LEMON-SPICED SHRIMP SALAD

SERVES 4

Antioxidants: tomatoes, romaine, lemon juice, shallots, avocados, black pepper

S/C Value = 4/2

2 cups tomatoes, sliced
3 Tbsp. lemon juice
3 Tbsp. shallots, diced
2 avocados, chopped
16 oz. cooked shrimp (about 30–40 shrimp), tails removed
2 cups romaine lettuce
Salt and pepper, to taste
2 small sourdough rolls
Butter, for serving

1. Mix tomato, lemon juice, shallots, avocado, and shrimp in a large salad bowl; season with salt and pepper, to taste. Divide romaine among 4 plates, and top with shrimp salad.

2. Serve each salad with half of a sourdough roll and some butter.

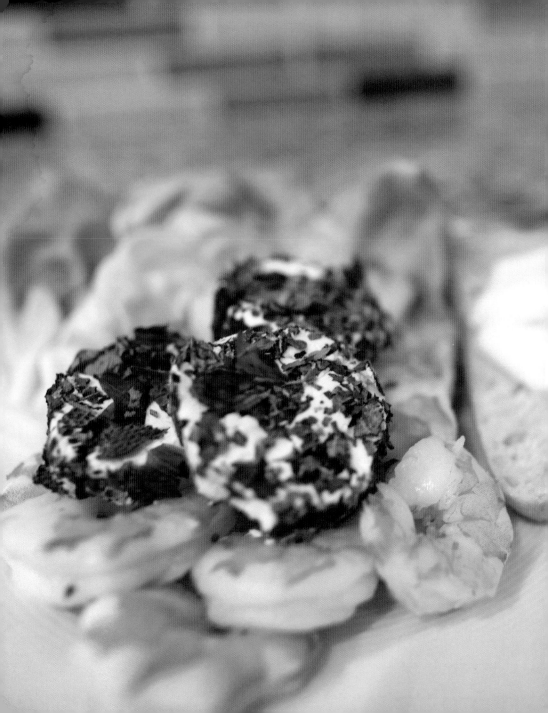

GOAT CHEESE AND SHRIMP SALAD

SERVES 4

Antioxidants: oregano, sage, basil, lemon juice, black pepper, thyme

S/C Value = 0/0

1 Tbsp. thyme
1 Tbsp. oregano
1 sage leaf, chopped
1 basil leaf, chopped
1 (6 oz.) log fresh goat cheese
1 Tbsp. lemon juice
8 oz. cooked shrimp (about 15–20 shrimp)
2 cups butter lettuce
Salt and pepper, to taste

1. Mix thyme, oregano, sage, and basil in a bowl. Roll goat cheese in the mixture; slice log into 1"-thick pieces. Place lemon juice in a bowl and toss shrimp in it; season with salt and pepper, to taste. Place lettuce on plates and top with herb-crusted goat cheese and shrimp.

2. Sprinkle with remaining herbs before serving.

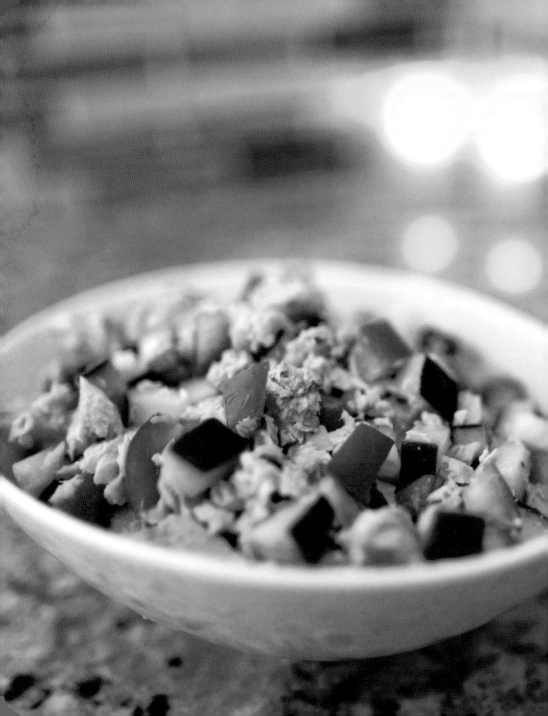

CRUNCHY SALMON SALAD

SERVES 4

Antioxidants: salmon, scallions, lemon juice, extra-virgin olive oil, black pepper, red bell pepper

S/C Value = 4/1

24 oz. canned salmon

2 cucumbers, chopped

1 red bell pepper, chopped

4 scallions, chopped

2 Tbsp. lemon juice

2 Tbsp. extra-virgin olive oil

Salt and pepper, to taste

1. Using a fork, flake salmon into a large salad bowl; add cucumber, red bell pepper, and scallions. In a small bowl, mix lemon juice and olive oil. Add lemon juice and olive oil to salad and toss to coat; season with salt and pepper, to taste.

2. Divide salad into four portions and serve.

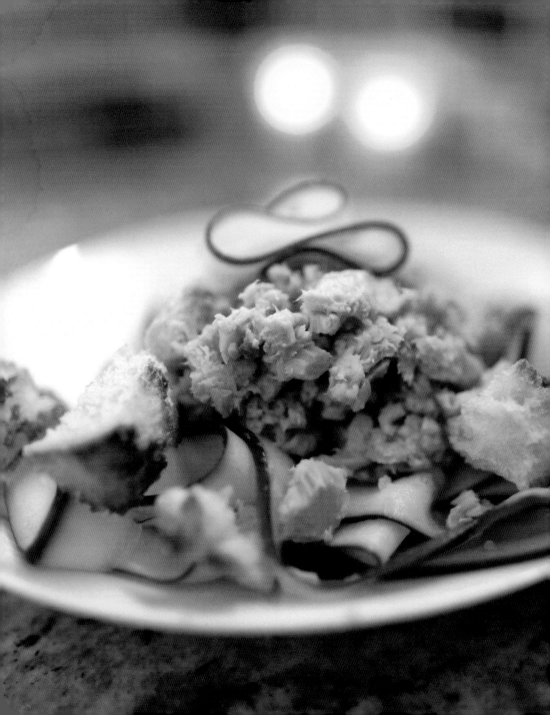

SALMON AND SOURDOUGH SALAD

SERVES 4

Antioxidants: salmon, extra-virgin olive oil, black pepper

S/C Value = 1/2

Half of (1 lb.) sourdough loaf, stale
18 oz. canned salmon
1 zucchini
2 Tbsp. extra-virgin olive oil
Salt and pepper, to taste

1. Cut crusts off of bread and tear into bite-sized pieces; place in a toaster oven and toast until just starting to brown. Using a fork, flake salmon into a large salad bowl. Cut zucchini in half lengthwise; using a peeler, make long, thin strips from each half. Add zucchini, toasted sourdough, and olive oil to salmon and toss to coat.

2. Season with salt and pepper, to taste, before serving.

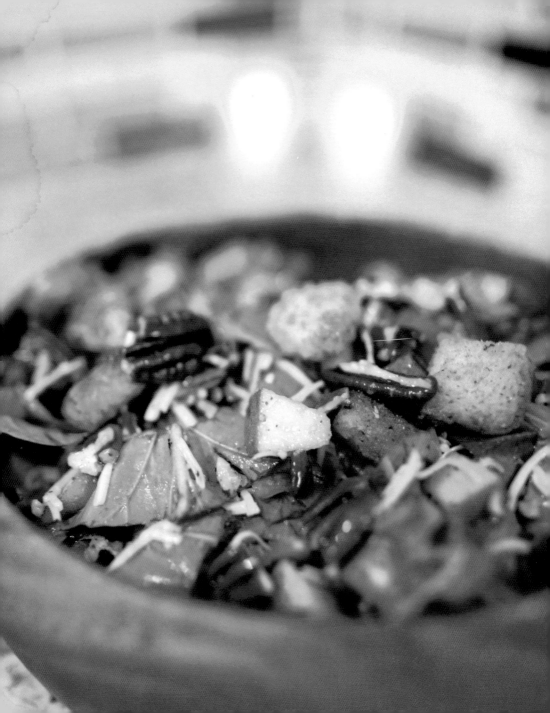

JUICY PEAR AND PECAN SALAD

SERVES 4

Antioxidants: spinach, pear, pecans

S/C Value = 5/1

4 cups spinach
½ pear, diced
1 cup pecans, chopped
1 cup mozzarella, grated
¼ cup Newman's Own Balsamic Vinaigrette
1 cup croutons

1. Mix spinach, pear, pecans, and mozzarella in a large salad bowl.
Toss with balsamic vinaigrette.

2. Serve salad topped with croutons.

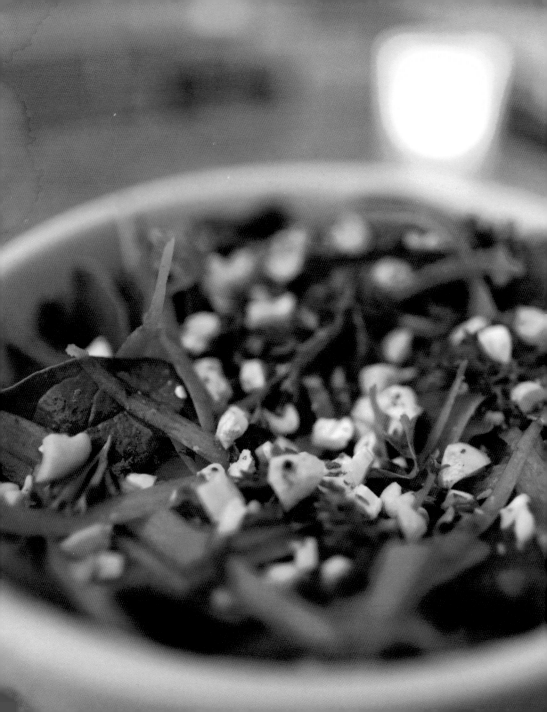

CRUNCHY CARROT AND CASHEW SALAD

SERVES 4

Antioxidants: carrots, spinach, parsley, cinnamon, extra-virgin olive oil, black pepper, cashews

S/C Value = 4/1

3 carrots

2 cups baby spinach

1 cup cashews, chopped

¼ cup fresh parsley, chopped

2 Tbsp. lime juice

2 Tbsp. extra-virgin olive oil

Salt and pepper, to taste

Cinnamon, to taste

1. With a peeler, create long, thin strands of carrot; mix with spinach, cashews, and parsley in a large salad bowl. Mix lime juice and olive oil in a small bowl; add to salad and toss to coat. Season with salt and pepper, to taste.

2. Sprinkle with cinnamon before serving.

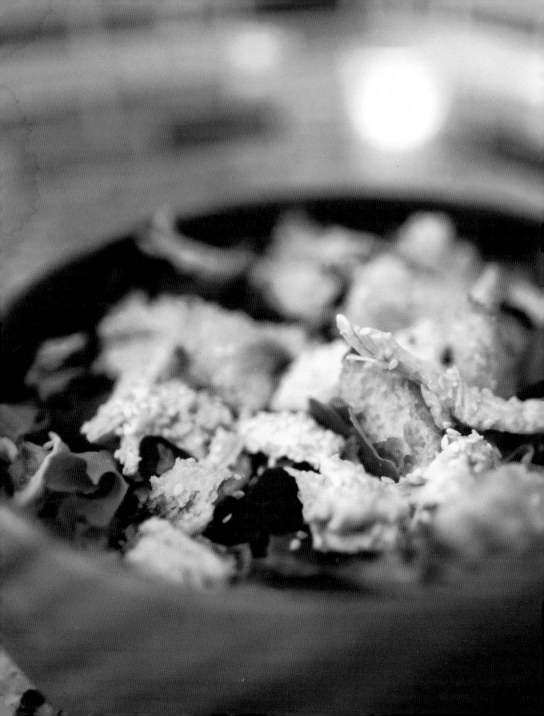

TANGY SESAME SOURDOUGH CHICKEN SALAD

SERVES 4

Antioxidants: red wine vinegar, sesame seeds, extra-virgin olive oil, black pepper, mixed greens

S/C Value = 1/2

Half of (1 lb.) sourdough loaf, stale
2 Tbsp. red wine vinegar
1 Tbsp. mustard
4 handfuls of meat from a rotisserie chicken
¼ cup sesame seeds
2 cups mixed greens
2 Tbsp. extra-virgin olive oil
Salt and pepper, to taste

1. Cut crusts off of bread and tear into bite-sized pieces; place in a toaster oven and toast until just starting to brown. Mix vinegar, mustard, and olive oil in a large salad bowl. Add toasted sourdough, chicken, sesame seeds, and mixed greens; toss.

2. Season with salt and pepper, to taste, before serving.

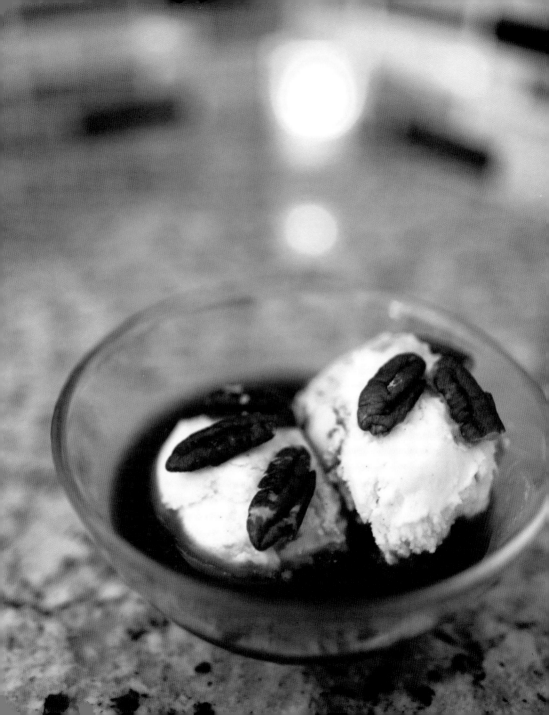

VANILLA, PECAN, AND ESPRESSO SUNDAE

SERVES 4

Antioxidants: espresso, pecans, cinnamon

S/C Value = 1/1

1 cup Clemmy's Vanilla Bean ice cream
4 shots espresso
1 cup pecans
Cinnamon, for serving

1. Scoop ice cream into 4 small dishes; pour one shot of espresso over each. (Be sure not to pour espresso onto ice cream until ready to serve, as it will melt very quickly.)

2. Sprinkle pecans and cinnamon on top before serving.

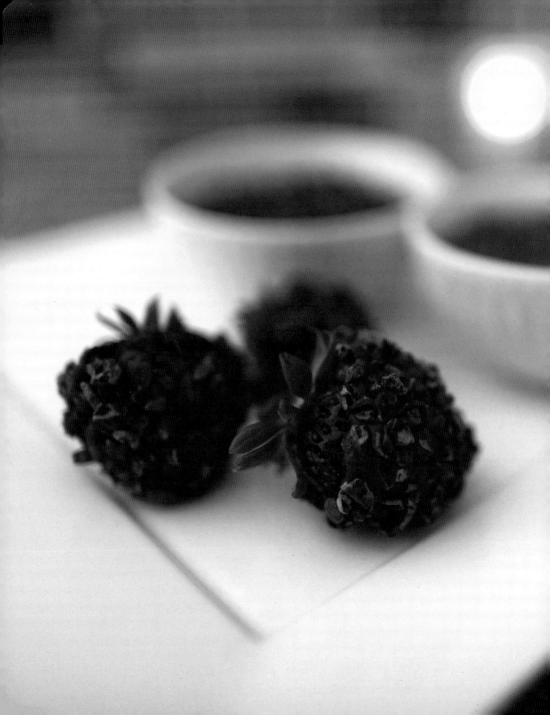

CREAMY PEANUT BUTTER–COVERED STRAWBERRIES

MAKES 12 STRAWBERRIES

Antioxidants: strawberries, cacao nibs

S/C Value = 4/1

12 strawberries
2 Tbsp. whipping cream
¼ cup peanut butter
½ cup cacao nibs

1. Mix peanut butter and whipping cream in a microwave-safe bowl. Microwave, stirring periodically, for 30 seconds, or until smooth; remove from microwave. Dip each strawberry into mixture. Place cacao nibs on a plate; roll each strawberry in them. Place completed strawberries on lightly greased wax paper.

2. Allow to sit for 15 minutes before serving with extra peanut butter cream.

GLACÉAU
vitaminwater
Zero
naturally sweetened

squeezed (8 key nutrients from a · zinc)

...etable flavored + other natural flavors

SWEET LEMONADE DREAM BARS

SERVES 4

Antioxidant: lemon juice

S/C Value = 1/1

½ cup half-and-half
½ cup whipping cream
1 cup Vitaminwater Zero Squeezed (lemonade flavor)
2 Tbsp. lemon juice

1. Mix all ingredients together in a bowl with a spout (such as a mixing cup). Pour into Popsicle mold; freeze for at least 4 hours.

2. Serve cold.

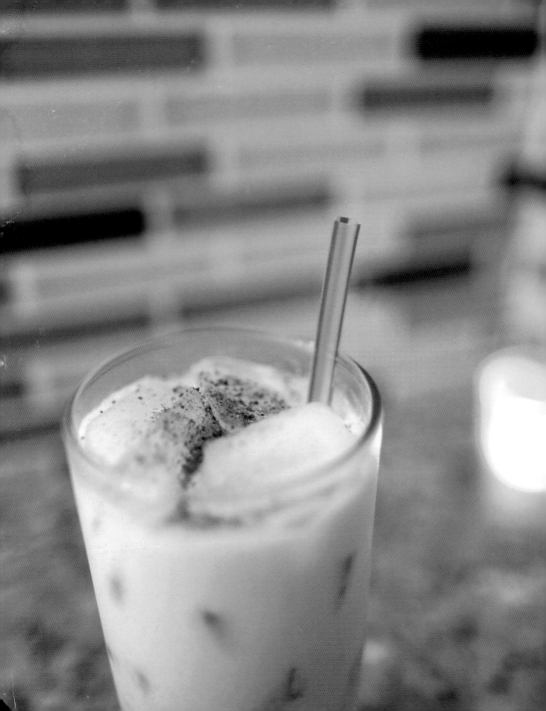

SWEET VANILLA CREAM BOURBON

SERVES 4

Antioxidants: cinnamon, nutmeg, almond milk

S/C Value = 0/0

2½ cups unsweetened almond milk, vanilla flavor
1½ cups half-and-half
1 cup bourbon
8 packets stevia
3 Tbsp. vanilla extract
Cinnamon, for serving
Nutmeg, for serving

1. Pour almond milk, half-and-half, and bourbon into a large pitcher; add stevia and vanilla extract and stir. Serve on the rocks or freeze until slushy (about 3 hours).

2. Sprinkle with cinnamon and nutmeg before serving.

Fat-Melting Carb Swap™
Products

Now that I've revealed the truth about hidden sugar, it's time to completely bust the myth that popular antioxidant-rich products are healthy. They're not. I'm about to show you exactly how much sugar is in many of these products and give you tasty alternatives that will help you age less. That's why I consider this chapter nothing short of magical.

As your coach, I will always recommend preparing a fresh meal with whole foods rich in antioxidants for the absolute best results, rather than having you rely on prepared products. However, I do understand that life can be hectic, and I want you to be aware of your options. If your cupboards and refrigerator contain some of the items considered Age More, I encourage you to start swapping them out gradually with the Age Less products I recommend. The following product categories include staples like breads, milk alternatives, and condiments; as well as snacks, teas, and gum to keep you satisfied. As with the recipes featured in the last chapter, all the S/C Values for the items here are based upon one serving size as listed on the food packaging.

Before your next visit to the grocery store, review this chapter. Simply making a few swaps can yield major results on your waistline, your youthfulness, your energy level, and your overall health. With these products in addition to the recipes in Chapter 4, you will feel lighter and rejuvenated in just two weeks!

Liquid Sweeteners

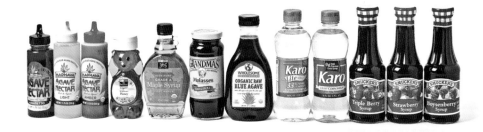

AGE MORE

1. Madhava Agave Nectar Amaretto: 15/1
2. Madhava Agave Nectar Light: 16/1
3. Madhava Agave Nectar Amber: 16/1
4. 365 Everyday Value Organic Wildflower Honey: 17/1
5. 365 Everyday Value Organic 100% Pure Grade A Maple Syrup Light Amber: 53/3
6. Grandma's Original Molasses: 14/1
7. Wholesome Sweeteners Organic Raw Blue Agave: 16/1
8. Karo Lite Syrup: 7/1
9. Karo Light Corn Syrup with Real Vanilla: 10/2
10. Smucker's Triple Berry Syrup: 44/3
11. Smucker's Strawberry Syrup: 44/3
12. Smucker's Boysenberry Syrup: 44/3

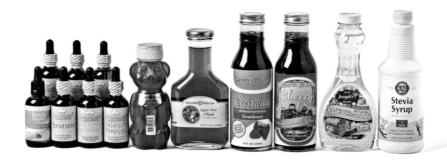

1. 365 Everyday Value Stevia Extract Liquid: 0/0
2. SweetLeaf Liquid Stevia Cinnamon: 0/0
3. SweetLeaf Liquid Stevia Lemon Drop: 0/0
4. SweetLeaf Liquid Stevia Valencia Orange: 0/0
5. SweetLeaf Liquid Stevia Chocolate: 0/0
6. SweetLeaf Liquid Stevia Vanilla Crème: 0/0
7. SweetLeaf Liquid Stevia Peppermint: 0/0
8. Nature's Hollow Sugar Free Honey Substitute: 0/1
9. Nature's Hollow Sugar Free Maple Flavored Syrup: 0/1
10. Nature's Flavors Erythritol Strawberry: 0/1
11. Nature's Flavors Cherry Flavored Syrup: 0/1
12. Joseph's All Natural Maltitol Sweetener: 0/1
13. KAL Stevia Syrup: 0/1

Powdered Sweeteners

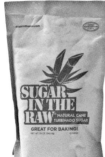
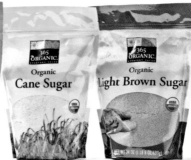
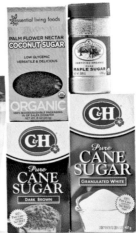

AGE MORE

1. Sugar In The Raw Natural Cane Turbinado Sugar: 4/0
2. 365 Everyday Value Organic Cane Sugar: 4/0
3. 365 Everyday Value Organic Light Brown Sugar: 4/0
4. C & H Pure Cane Sugar Dark Brown: 4/0
5. C & H Pure Cane Sugar Granulated White: 4/0
6. Essential Living Foods Palm Flower Nectar Coconut Sugar: 24/2
7. Shady Maple Farms Pure Maple Sugar: 4/0

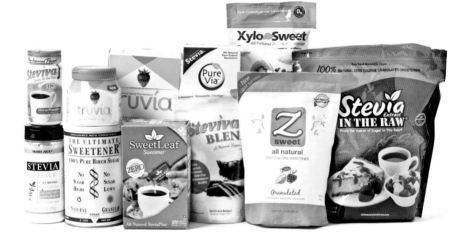

1. Trader Joe's Stevia Extract: 0/0
2. The Ultimate Sweetener 100% Pure Birch Sugar: 0/0
3. SweetLeaf Sweetener: 0/0
4. Steviva Blend: 0/0
5. ZSweet All Natural Zero Calorie Sweetener: 0/0
6. Stevia Extract In The Raw: 0/0
7. Steviva Stevia Powder: 0/0
8. Scoopable Truvia: 0/0
9. Truvia Packets: 0/0
10. Stevia Pure Via: 0/0
11. XyloSweet All Natural Xylitol Sweetner: 0/0

Cereal

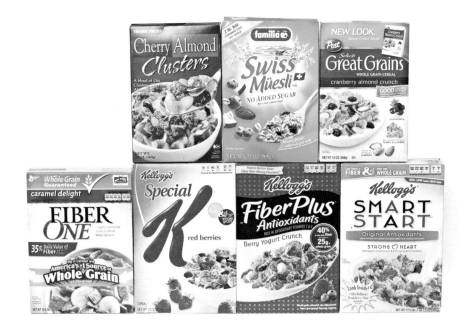

AGE MORE

1. Fiber One Caramel Delight: 10/3
2. Kellogg's Special K Red Berries: 9/2
3. Kellogg's FiberPlus Antioxidants Berry Yogurt Crunch: 12/3
4. Kellogg's Smart Start Original Antioxidants: 14/3
5. Trader Joe's Cherry Almond Clusters: 18/3
6. Familia Swiss Muesli: 7/3
7. Post Selects Great Grains Cranberry Almond Crunch: 13/2

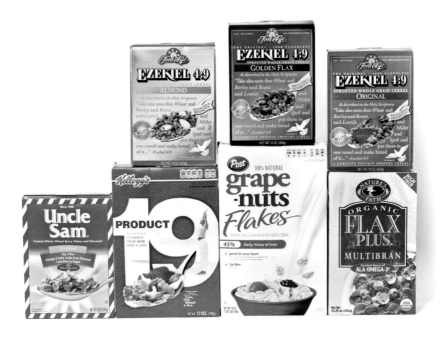

AGE LESS

1. Uncle Sam Original: 0/2
2. Kellogg's Product 19: 4/2
3. Post Grape-Nuts Flakes: 4/2
4. Nature's Path Organic Flax Plus Multibran Flakes: 4/2
5. Ezekiel 4:9 Almond: 0/2
6. Ezekiel 4:9 Golden Flax: 0/2
7. Ezekiel 4:9 Original: 0/2

Breakfast Bars

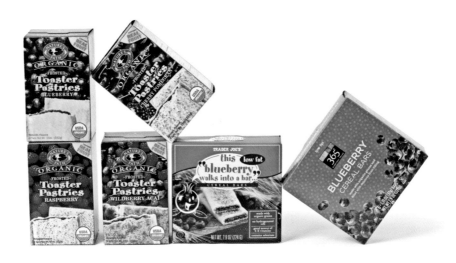

AGE MORE

1. Nature's Path Organic Frosted Raspberry Toaster Pastries: 18/2
2. Nature's Path Organic Frosted Wildberry Acai Toaster Pastries: 18/2
3. Trader Joe's Low Fat This "Blueberry Walks Into a Bar . . ." Cereal Bars: 16/2
4. 365 Everyday Value Blueberry Cereal Bars: 17/2
5. Nature's Path Organic Frosted Blueberry Toaster Pastries: 20/2
6. Nature's Path Organic Frosted Cherry Pomegranate Toaster Pastries: 17/2

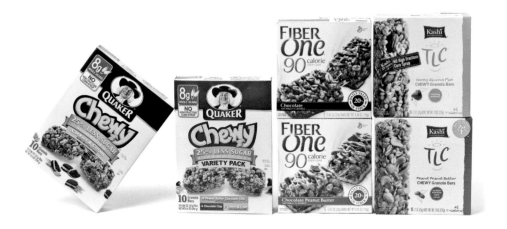

AGE LESS

1. Quaker Chewy Cookies & Cream 25% Less Sugar: 5/1
2. Quaker Chewy Variety Pack 25% Less Sugar: 5/1
3. Fiber One Chocolate Peanut Butter 90 Calorie Chewy Bars: 5/1
4. Kashi TLC Peanut Peanut Butter Chewy Granola Bars: 5/1
5. Fiber One Chocolate 90 Calorie Chewy Bars: 5/1
6. Kashi TLC Honey Almond Flax Chewy Granola Bars: 5/1

Bread

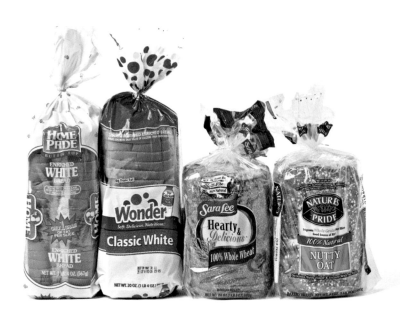

AGE MORE

1. Home Pride Enriched White Bread: 3/1
2. Wonder Classic White: 4/2
3. Sara Lee Hearty & Delicious 100% Whole Wheat: 5/2
4. Nature's Pride 100% Natural Nutty Oat: 4/1

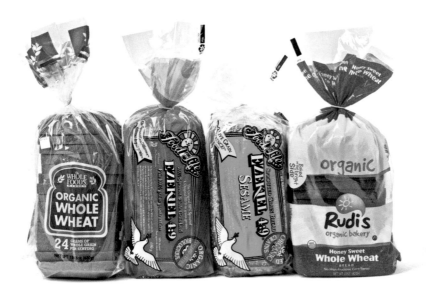

AGE LESS

1. Whole Foods Organic Whole Wheat: 0/2
2. Ezekiel 4:9 100% Sprouted Whole Grain Loaf: 0/1
3. Ezekiel 4:9 Sesame Bread: 0/1
4. Rudi's Organic Bakery Honey Sweet Whole Wheat Bread: 2/1

Buns

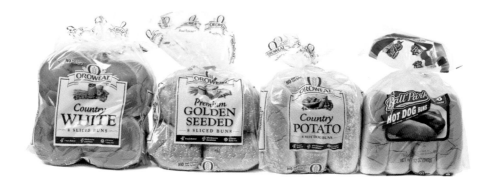

AGE MORE

1. Oroweat Country White Sliced Buns: 7/2
2. Oroweat Premium Golden Seeded Sliced Buns: 5/2
3. Oroweat Country Potato Hot Dog Buns: 6/2
4. Ball Park Hot Dog Buns: 4/2

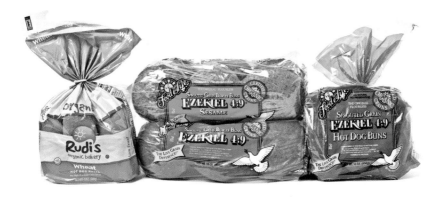

AGE LESS

1. Rudi's Organic Bakery Wheat Hot Dog Rolls: 3/2
2. Ezekiel 4:9 Sprouted Grain Burger Buns: 0/2
3. Ezekiel 4:9 Sesame Sprouted Grain Burger Buns: 0/2
4. Ezekiel 4:9 Sprouted Grain Hot Dog Buns: 0/2

Almond & Soy Products

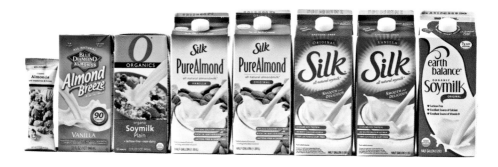

AGE MORE

1. Starbucks Glazed Almonds with Cranberries & Honey: 9/1
2. Blue Diamond Almond Breeze Vanilla: 15/1
3. O Organics Organic Soymilk Plain: 6/1
4. Silk Pure Almond Vanilla Almond Milk: 15/1
5. Silk Pure Almond Original Almond Milk: 7/1
6. Silk Original Soymilk: 6/1
7. Silk Vanilla Soymilk: 8/1
8. Earth Balance Organic Soymilk Original: 7/1

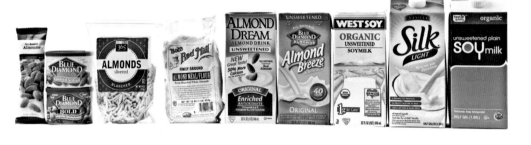

AGE LESS

1. Starbucks Dry-Roasted Almonds: 1/1
2. Blue Diamond Bold Jalapeño Smokehouse Almonds: 1/1
3. Blue Diamond Roasted Salted Blanched Almonds: 1/1
4. 365 Everyday Value Slivered Blanched Almonds: 1/1
5. Bob's Red Mill Finely Ground Almond Meal Flour: 1/1
6. Almond Dream Unsweetened Original Almond Drink: 0/0
7. Blue Diamond Almond Breeze Unsweetened Original: 0/0
8. Westsoy Organic Unsweetened Soymilk: 1/1
9. Silk Light Vanilla Soymilk: 5/1
10. Fresh & Easy Organic Unsweetened Plain Soymilk: 1/0

Coconut Products

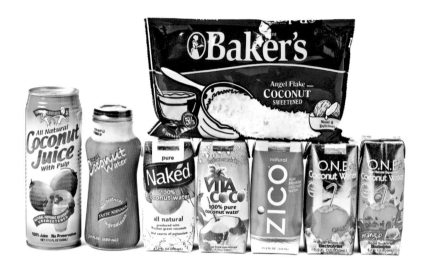

AGE MORE

1. Amy & Brian All Natural Coconut Juice with Pulp: 10/1
2. Taste Nirvana Real Coconut Water: 9/1
3. Naked 100% Coconut Water: 11/1
4. Vita Coco 100% Pure Coconut Water: 15/1
5. ZICO Pure Premium Coconut Water: 14/1
6. O.N.E. Coconut Water: 14/1
7. O.N.E. Coconut Water with a Splash of Mango: 16/1
8. Baker's Angel Flake Coconut Sweetened: 5/1

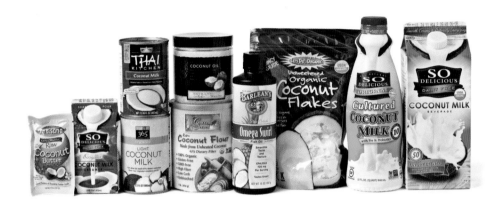

AGE LESS

1. Artisana Raw Coconut Butter: 2/1
2. So Delicious Coconut Milk Creamer: 1/0
3. 365 Everyday Value Organic Light Coconut Milk: 0/0
4. Coconut Secret Raw Coconut Flour: 1/1
5. Barlean's Piña Colada Omega Swirl: 0/0
6. Let's Do . . . Organic Unsweetened Organic Coconut Flakes: 1/0
7. So Delicious Original Cultured Coconut Milk: 3/1
8. So Delicious Unsweetened Coconut Milk: 0/0
9. Thai Kitchen Coconut Milk: 1/0
10. Ojio 100% Organic Coconut Oil: 0/0

Fruit Preserves

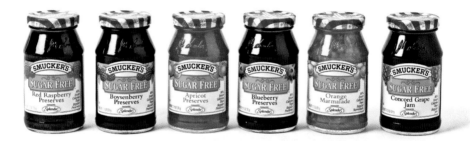

AGE MORE

1. Smucker's Sugar Free Red Raspberry Preserves: 0/1*
2. Smucker's Sugar Free Boysenberry Preserves: 0/1*
3. Smucker's Sugar Free Apricot Preserves: 0/1*
4. Smucker's Sugar Free Blueberry Preserves: 0/1*
5. Smucker's Sugar Free Orange Marmalade: 0/1*
6. Smucker's Sugar Free Concord Grape Jam: 0/1*

*contains sucralose, an artificial sweetener that I strongly advise against

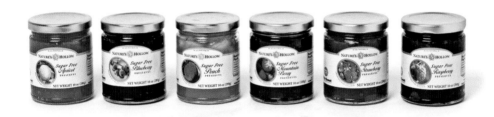

AGE LESS

1. Nature's Hollow Sugar Free Apricot Preserves: 0/1*
2. Nature's Hollow Sugar Free Blueberry Preserves: 0/1*
3. Nature's Hollow Sugar Free Peach Preserves: 0/1*
4. Nature's Hollow Sugar Free Mountain Berry Preserves: 0/1*
5. Nature's Hollow Sugar Free Strawberry Preserves: 0/1*
6. Nature's Hollow Sugar Free Raspberry Preserves: 0/1*

*contains xylitol, a sweetener extracted from the fibers of fruit and vegetables that does not cause blood-sugar spikes

Condiments

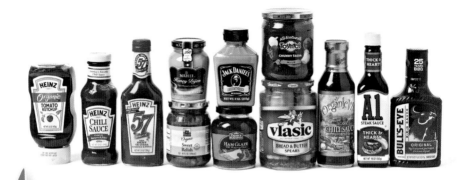

AGE MORE

1. Heinz Organic Tomato Ketchup: 4/1
2. Heinz Chili Sauce: 3/1
3. Heinz 57 Sauce: 4/1
4. 365 Everyday Value Organic Sweet Relish: 4/0
5. Crosse & Blackwell Premium Ham Glaze with Montmorency Cherries: 5/1
6. Vlasic Bread & Butter Spears: 5/1
7. Organicville Organic Chili Sauce: 4/1
8. A.1. Steak Sauce Thick & Hearty: 5/1
9. Bull's-Eye Original BBQ Sauce: 12/1
10. Maille Honey Dijon: 2/0
11. Jack Daniel's Honey Dijon Mustard: 2/0
12. Tostitos Mild Chunky Salsa: 2/0

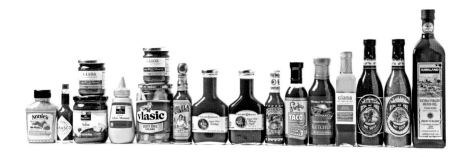

1. Annie's Naturals Organic Horseradish Mustard: 0/0
2. Tabasco Pepper Sauce: 0/0
3. 365 Everyday Value Organic Medium Salsa: 1/0
4. Giada de Laurentiis Genovese Basil Pesto: 0/0
5. 365 Everyday Value Organic Yellow Mustard: 0/0
6. Vlasic Zesty Dill Spears: 0/0
7. Giada de Laurentiis Sun-Dried Tomato: 2/0
8. Cholula Chili Garlic Hot Sauce: 0/0
9. Nature's Hollow Sugar Free Ketchup: 0/1
10. Nature's Hollow Sugar Free Hickory Maple BBQ Sauce: 0/1
11. Iguana Radioactive Atomic Pepper Sauce: 0/0
12. Frontera Gourmet Chipotle Garlic Taco Sauce with Roasted Tomato: 2/0
13. Westbrae Natural Unsweetened Ketchup: 0/0
14. Giada de Laurentiis Chile Dipping Oil: 0/0
15. Ring of Fire XX-Hot Habanero Hot Sauce: 0/0
16. Ring of Fire Tomatillo & Roasted Garlic Hot Sauce: 0/0
17. Kirkland Signature Extra Virgin Olive Oil: 0/0

*You'll notice that there are items with an S/C Value of 2/0 on both the Age More and Age Less sides. These items with an S/C Value of 2/0 are Age More because there are equivalent condiments with an S/C Value of 0/0, which are therefore better choices. The tomato sauce with an S/C Value of 2/0 is on the Age Less side because it is low in sugar for that type of condiment.

Dressings

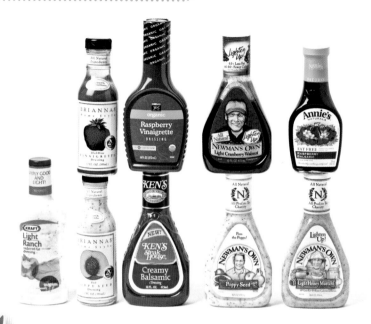

AGE MORE

1. Kraft Light Ranch Reduced Fat: 2/1
2. Briannas Poppy Seed Dressing: 7/1
3. Ken's Steak House Creamy Balsamic Dressing: 6/1
4. Newman's Own Poppy Seed: 5/1
5. Newman's Own Light Honey Mustard: 5/1
6. Briannas Blush Wine Vinaigrette Dressing: 14/1
7. 365 Everyday Value Organic Raspberry Vinaigrette: 4/1
8. Newman's Own Light Cranberry Walnut: 7/1
9. Annie's Naturals Fat Free Raspberry Balsamic Vinaigrette: 7/1

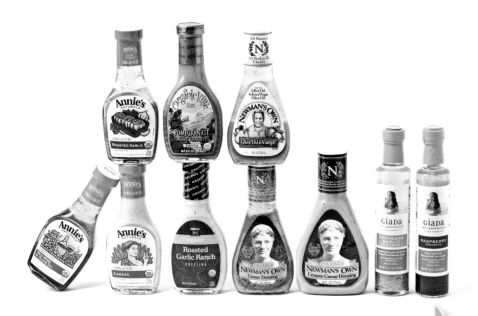

1. Annie's Naturals Organic Red Wine & Olive Oil Vinaigrette: 0/0
2. Annie's Naturals Organic Caesar Dressing: 2/0
3. 365 Everyday Value Organic Roasted Garlic Ranch: 0/0
4. Newman's Own Caesar Dressing: 1/0
5. Newman's Own Creamy Caesar Dressing: 0/0
6. Giada de Laurentiis Parmesan Garlic Vinaigrette: 0/0
7. Giada de Laurentiis Raspberry Vinaigrette: 2/0
8. Annie's Naturals Organic Roasted Garlic Vinaigrette: 2/0
9. Organicville Pomegranate Organic Vinaigrette: 2/0
10. Newman's Own Olive Oil & Vinegar: 1/0

Energy Bars

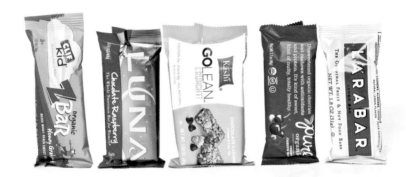

AGE MORE

1. Clif Kid Honey Graham Z Organic Bar: 10/2
2. Luna Chocolate Raspberry Bar: 13/2
3. Kashi Go Lean Crunchy! Chocolate Caramel: 14/2
4. Pure Organic Cherry Cashew Bar: 17/2
5. Larabar Lemon Bar: 22/2

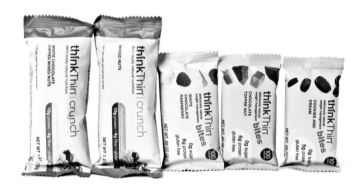

1. thinkThin Crunch White Chocolate Dipped Mixed Nuts: 3/1
2. thinkThin Crunch Mixed Nuts: 4/1
3. thinkThin White Chocolate Raspberry Bites: 0/1
4. thinkThin Chocolate Toffee Nut Bites: 0/1
5. thinkThin Cookies and Cream Bites: 0/1

Rice Snacks

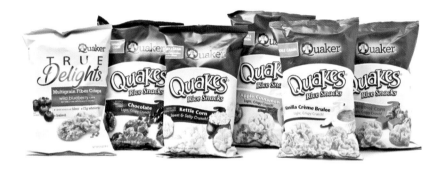

AGE MORE

1. Quaker Wild Blueberry True Delights: 6/2
2. Quaker Chocolate Quakes: 7/2
3. Quaker Kettle Corn Quakes: 7/2
4. Quaker Apple Cinnamon Quakes: 8/2
5. Quaker Vanilla Crème Brulée Quakes: 8/2
6. Quaker Caramel Corn Quakes: 9/2

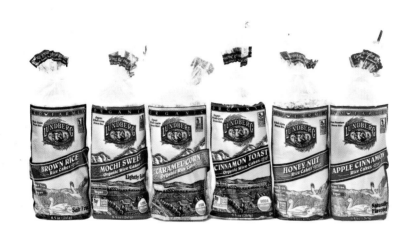

AGE LESS

1. Lundberg Brown Rice Rice Cakes: 0/1
2. Lundberg Mochi Sweet Organic Rice Cakes: 0/1
3. Lundberg Caramel Corn Organic Rice Cakes: 2/1
4. Lundberg Cinnamon Toast Organic Rice Cakes: 3/1
5. Lundberg Honey Nut Rice Cakes: 2/1
6. Lundberg Apple Cinnamon Rice Cakes: 2/1

Snacks

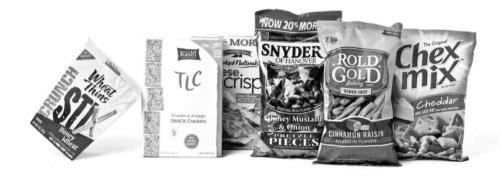

AGE MORE

1. Nabisco Wheat Thins Crunch Stix Honey Wheat: 5/2
2. Kashi TLC Toasted Asiago Snack Crackers: 2/2
3. Pepperidge Farm Baked Naturals Cheese Crisps Four Cheese: 3/1
4. Snyder's of Hanover Honey Mustard & Onion Pretzel Pieces: 3/1
5. Rold Gold Cinnamon Raisin Braided Pretzel Twists: 4/2
6. Chex Mix Cheddar: 3/2

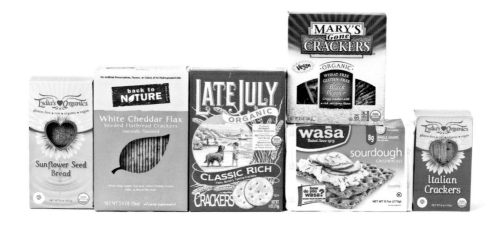

1. Lydia's Organics Sunflower Seed Bread: 0/1
2. Back to Nature White Cheddar Flax Seeded Flatbread Crackers: 2/1
3. Late July Organic Classic Rich Crackers: 2/1
4. Wasa Sourdough Crispbread: 0/1
5. Lydia's Organics Italian Crackers: 1/1
6. Mary's Gone Crackers Organic Black Pepper: 0/2

Cookies

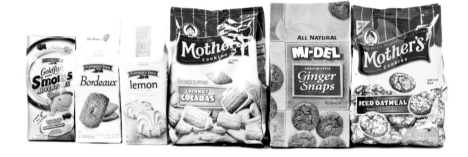

AGE MORE

1. Goldfish S'mores Adventures: 10/2
2. Pepperidge Farm Bordeaux Cookies: 12/1
3. Pepperidge Farm Lemon Cookies: 8/2
4. Mother's Cookies Coconut Cocadas: 9/2
5. Mi-Del Swedish Style Ginger Snaps: 11/2
6. Mother's Cookies Iced Oatmeal: 12/2

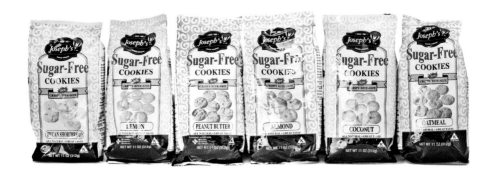

AGE LESS

1. Joseph's Sugar-Free Pecan Shortbread Cookies: 0/1

2. Joseph's Sugar-Free Lemon Cookies: 0/1

3. Joseph's Sugar-Free Peanut Butter Cookies: 0/1

4. Joseph's Sugar-Free Almond Cookies: 0/1

5. Joseph's Sugar-Free Coconut Cookies: 0/1

6. Joseph's Sugar-Free Oatmeal Cookies: 0/1

Gum & Candy

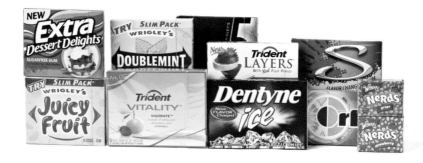

AGE MORE

1. Wrigley's Juicy Fruit: 2/0
2. Trident Vitality Vigorate: 0/0**
3. Dentyne Ice Arctic Chill: 0/0**
4. Orbit Maui Melon Mint Gum: 0/0**
5. Grape Nerds: 12/1
6. Strawberry Nerds: 12/1
7. Wrigley's Extra Dessert Delights Strawberry Shortcake Sugarfree Gum**: 0/0
8. Wrigley's Doublemint Gum: 2/0*
9 Wrigley's 5 Rain Gum: 0/0*
10. Trident Layers Wild Strawberry + Tangy Citrus: 0/0**
11. Stride Shift Gum: 0/0**

*contains aspartame, an artificial sweetener that I strongly advise against
**contains aspartame and sucralose, artificial sweeteners that I strongly advise against

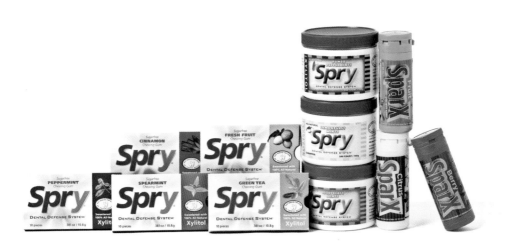

AGE LESS

1. Spry Sugarfree Peppermint Gum: 0/0*
2. Spry Sugarfree Spearmint Gum: 0/0*
3. Spry Sugarfree Green Tea Gum: 0/0*
4. Spry Berryblast Mints: 0/0*
5. Spry Lemonburst Mints: 0/0*
6. Spry Power Peppermints: 0/0*
7. Fruit Sparx: 0/0*
8. Citrus Sparx: 0/0*
9. Berry Sparx: 0/0*
10. Spry Sugarfree Cinnamon Gum: 0/0*
11. Spry Sugarfree Fresh Fruit Gum: 0/0*

*contains xylitol, a sweetener extracted from the fibers of fruit and vegetables that does not cause blood-sugar spikes.

Regular Coffee

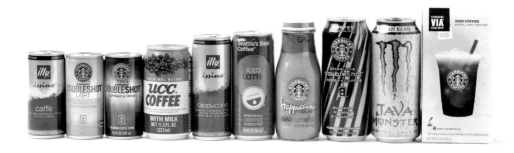

AGE MORE

1. Illy Issimo Caffè: 10/1
2. Starbucks Coffee Doubleshot Light Espresso & Cream: 5/1
3. Starbucks Coffee Doubleshot Espresso & Cream: 17/1
4. UCC Coffee Original Blend with Milk: 25/2
5. Illy Issimo Cappuccino: 18/1
6. Seattle's Best Coffee Iced Latte: 23/2
7. Starbucks Coffee Coffee Frappuccino: 32/2
8. Starbucks Coffee Doubleshot Energy + Coffee: 14/1
9. Java Monster Mean Bean: 16/1
10. Starbucks Via Ready Brew Iced Coffee: 11/1

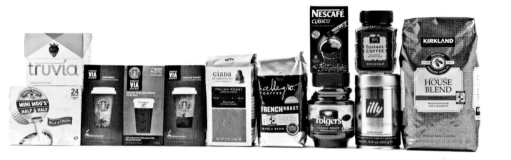

1. Land O Lakes Mini Moo's Half & Half: 0/0
2. Truvia Packet: 0/0
3. Starbucks Via Ready Brew Colombia Medium: 0/0
4. Starbucks Via Ready Brew Decaf Italian Roast: 0/0
5. Starbucks Via Ready Brew Italian Roast Extra Bold: 0/0
6. Giada de Laurentiis Italian Roast Ground Coffee: 0/0
7. Allegro Coffee Organic French Roast: 0/0
8. Folgers Classic Roast: 0/0
9. Illy Dark Roast Ground Coffee: 0/0
10. Kirkland Signature Medium Roast House Blend: 0/0
11. Nescafé Clásico: 0/0
12. 365 Everyday Value Instant Coffee: 0/0

Chocolate & Vanilla Coffee

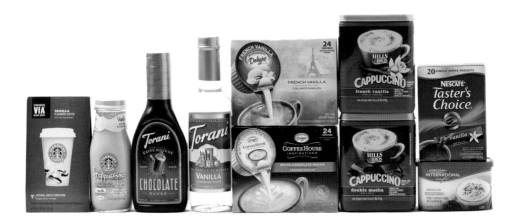

AGE MORE

1. Starbucks Via Ready Brew Vanilla Flavored Single-Serve Packets: 13/1
2. Starbucks Coffee Bottled Vanilla Light Frappuccino: 11/1
3. Torani Chocolate Sauce: 20/2
4. Torani Vanilla Flavoring Syrup: 16/1
5. International Delight French Vanilla Creamer Singles: 6/1
6. International Delight White Chocolate Mocha Creamer Singles: 5/1
7. Hills Bros. French Vanilla Cappuccino: 15/1
8. Hills Bros. Double Mocha Cappuccino: 15/1
9. Nescafé Taster's Choice Vanilla Single-Serve Packet: 0/0*
10. Maxwell House International Café Mocha Latte: 9/1

*contains aspartame, an artificial sweetener that I strongly advise against.

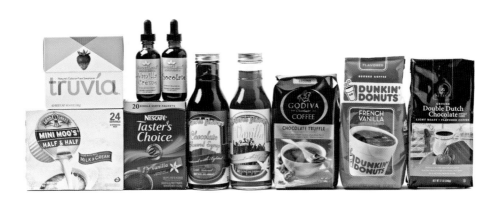

AGE LESS

1. Land O Lakes Mini Moo's Half & Half: 0/0
2. Truvia Packet: 0/0
3. Nescafé Taster's Choice Vanilla Single-Serve Packets: 0/0
4. Nature's Flavors Chocolate Flavored Syrup: 0/1
5. Nature's Flavors Vanilla Flavored Syrup: 0/0
6. Godiva Chocolate Truffle Ground Coffee: 0/0
7. Dunkin' Donuts French Vanilla Ground Coffee: 0/0
8. Safeway Select Ground Double Dutch Chocolate: 0/0
9. SweetLeaf Liquid Stevia Vanilla Crème: 0/0
10. SweetLeaf Liquid Stevia Chocolate: 0/0

Caramel Coffee

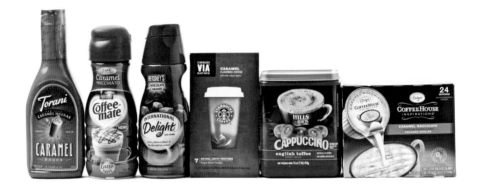

AGE MORE

1. Torani Caramel Sauce: 14/2
2. Nestlé Coffee-Mate Caramel Macchiato: 5/1
3. International Delight Hershey's Chocolate Caramel Creamer: 6/1
4. Starbucks Via Ready Brew Caramel Flavored Coffee Single-Serve Packets: 13/1
5. Hills Bros. English Toffee Cappuccino: 15/1
6. International Delight CoffeeHouse Inspirations Caramel Macchiato Creamer Singles: 5/1

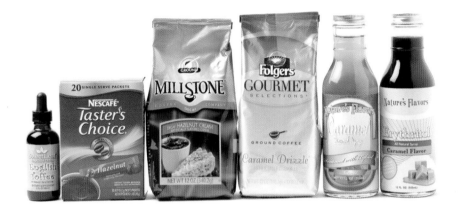

1. SweetLeaf Liquid Stevia English Toffee: 0/0
2. Nescafé Taster's Choice Hazelnut Single Serve Packets: 0/0
3. Millstone Decaf Hazelnut Cream Ground Coffee: 0/0
4. Folgers Gourmet Caramel Drizzle Ground Coffee: 0/0
5. Nature's Flavors Caramel Flavored Syrup: 0/0
6. Nature's Flavors Erythritol Caramel Flavor: 0/1

Vitaminwater

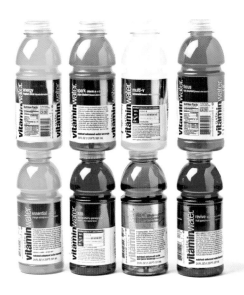

AGE MORE

1. Vitaminwater Essential: 13/1
2. Vitaminwater XXX: 13/1
3. Vitaminwater Stur-D: 9/1
4. Vitaminwater Revive: 13/1
5. Vitaminwater Energy: 13/1
6. Vitaminwater Spark: 13/1
7. Vitaminwater Multi-V: 13/1
8. Vitaminwater Focus: 13/1

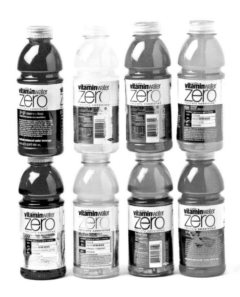

AGE LESS

1. Vitaminwater Zero XXX: 0/0
2. Vitaminwater Zero Rhythm: 0/0
3. Vitaminwater Zero Mega-C: 0/0
4. Vitaminwater Zero Drive: 0/0
5. Vitaminwater Zero Go-Go: 0/0
6. Vitaminwater Zero Squeezed: 0/0
7. Vitaminwater Zero Glow: 0/0
8. Vitaminwater Zero Rise: 0/0

SoBe Drinks

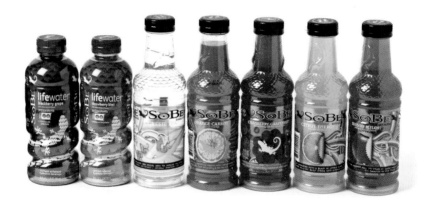

AGE MORE

1. SoBe Lifewater Blackberry Grape: 9/1
2. SoBe Lifewater Strawberry Kiwi: 10/1
3. SoBe Energize Green: 25/2
4. SoBe Vita-Boom Orange Carrot: 23/2
5. SoBe Vita-Boom Cranberry Grapefruit: 26/2
6. SoBe Energize Citrus Energy: 27/2
7. SoBe Energize Mango Melon: 29/2

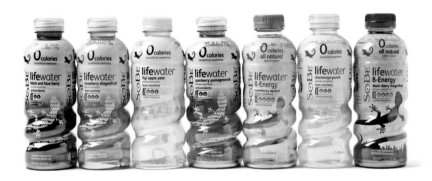

AGE LESS

1. SoBe Lifewater Black and Blue Berry: 0/1
2. SoBe Lifewater Strawberry Dragonfruit: 0/1
3. SoBe Lifewater Fuji Apple Pear: 0/1
4. SoBe Lifewater Yumberry Pomegranate: 0/1
5. SoBe Lifewater B-Energy Strawberry Apricot: 0/1
6. SoBe Lifewater Cherimoya Punch: 0/1
7. SoBe Lifewater B-Energy Black Cherry Dragonfruit: 0/1

Flavored Beverages

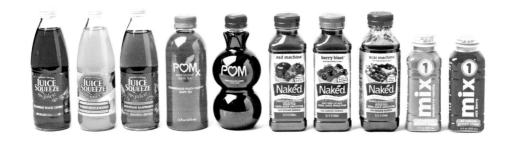

AGE MORE

1. Crystal Geyser Cranberry Black Cherry Juice Squeeze: 33/2
2. Crystal Geyser Passion Fruit & Mango Juice Squeeze: 27/2
3. Crystal Geyser Mountain Raspberry Juice Squeeze: 29/2
4. PomX Pomegranate Peach Passion White Tea: 17/1
5. Pom Wonderful Pomegranate Cherry: 29/2
6. Naked Red Machine: 25/2
7. Naked Berry Blast: 26/2
8. Naked Acai Machine: 24/2
9. Mix1 Blueberry-Vanilla All-Natural Protein Shake: 22/2
10. Mix1 Mix Berry All-Natural Protein Shake: 22/2

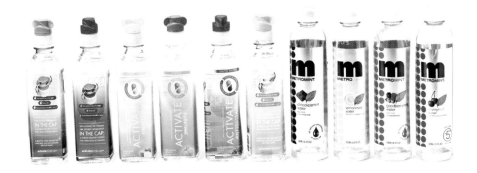

AGE LESS

1. Activate Antioxidant Blueberry Pomegranate: 0/0
2. Activate Vitamin Fruit Punch: 0/0
3. Activate Energy Lemon Lime: 0/0
4. Activate Immunity Orange: 0/0
5. Activate Antioxidant Exotic Berry: 0/0
6. Activate Multivitamin Lulo Pear: 0/0
7. Metromint Chocolatemint Water: 0/0
8. Metromint Lemonmint Water: 0/0
9. Metromint Goodberrymint Water: 0/0
10. Metromint Cherrymint Water: 0/0

Flavored Tea

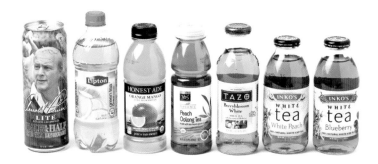

AGE MORE

1. Arnold Palmer Lite Half & Half: 13/1
2. Lipton Citrus Flavored Green Tea: 0/0*
3. Honest Ade Orange Mango: 12/1
4. 365 Everyday Value Organic Peach Oolong Tea: 8/1
5. Tazo Berryblossom White Tea: 8/1
6. Inko's White Peach Tea: 7/1
7. Inko's Blueberry White Tea: 7/1

*contains aspartame, an artificial sweetener that I strongly advise against

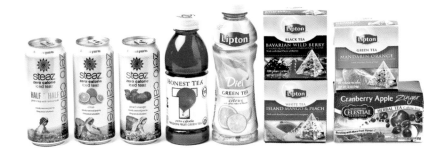

AGE LESS

1. Steaz Half & Half: 0/0
2. Steaz Citrus: 0/0
3. Steaz Peach Mango: 0/0
4. Honest Tea Passion Fruit: 0/0
5. Lipton Unsweetened Lemon Green Tea: 0/0
6. Lipton Island Mango & Peach: 0/0
7. Celestial Cranberry Apple Zinger: 0/0
8. Lipton Bavarian Wild Berry: 0/0
9. Lipton Mandarin Orange: 0/0

Green Tea

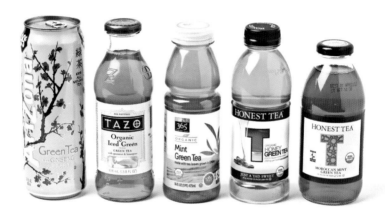

AGE MORE

1. Arizona Green Tea with Ginseng and Honey: 17/1
2. Tazo Organic Iced Green Tea: 18/1
3. 365 Everyday Value Organic Mint Green Tea: 8/1
4. Honest Tea Organic Honey Green Tea: 9/1
5. Honest Tea Moroccan Mint Green Tea: 5/1

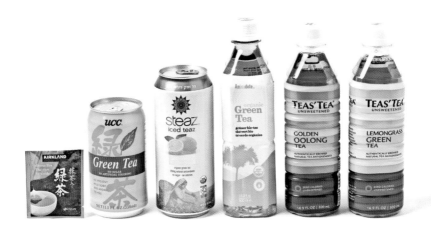

AGE LESS

1. Kirkland Signature Ito En Green Tea: 0/0
2. UCC Green Tea: 0/0
3. Steaz Iced Teaz Unsweetened Lemon: 0/0
4. Anteadote Organic Green Tea: 0/0
5. Teas'Tea Unsweetened Golden Oolong Tea: 0/0
6. Teas'Tea Unsweetened Lemongrass Green Tea: 0/0

Black & White Tea

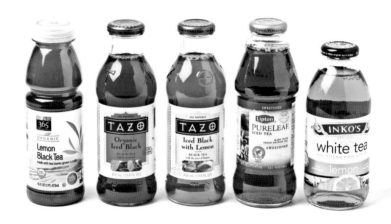

AGE MORE

1. 365 Everyday Value Organic Lemon Black Tea: 8/1
2. Tazo Organic Iced Black Tea: 9/1
3. Tazo Iced Black with Lemon: 20/1
4. Lipton Pureleaf Sweetened Iced Tea: 18/1
5. Inko's White Tea Lemon: 7/1

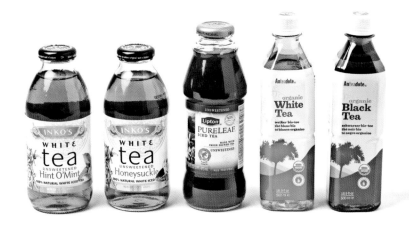

AGE LESS

1. Inko's White Tea Unsweetened Hint O'Mint: 0/0
2. Inko's White Tea Unsweetened Honeysuckle: 0/0
3. Lipton Pureleaf Unsweetened Iced Tea: 0/0
4. Anteadote Organic White Tea: 0/0
5. Anteadote Organic Black Tea: 0/0

Sparkling Beverages

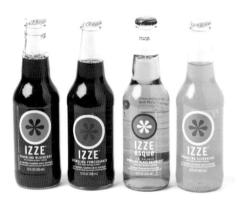

AGE MORE

1. IZZE Sparkling Blueberry: 31/2
2. IZZE Sparkling Pomegranate: 26/2
3. IZZE Esque Sparkling Black Raspberry: 11/1
4. IZZE Sparkling Clementine: 27/2

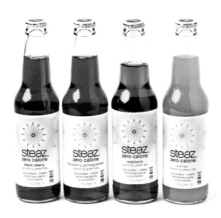

AGE LESS

1. Steaz Black Cherry Sparkling Green Tea: 0/0
2. Steaz Blueberry Pomegranate Sparkling Green Tea: 0/0
3. Steaz Raspberry Sparkling Green Tea: 0/0
4. Steaz Orange Sparkling Green Tea: 0/0

Protein Drinks

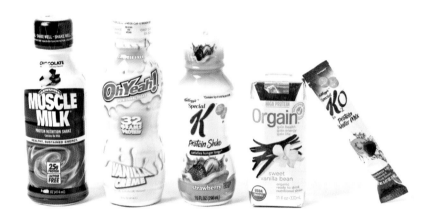

AGE MORE

1. Muscle Milk Chocolate Protein Nutrition Shake: 3/1
2. OhYeah! Vanilla Crème Nutritional Shake: 3/0
3. Special K Strawberry Protein Shake: 18/2
4. Orgain Sweet Vanilla Bean: 13/2
5. Special K_2O Strawberry Kiwi Protein Water Mix: 0/1*

*contains sucralose, an artificial sweetener that I strongly advise against

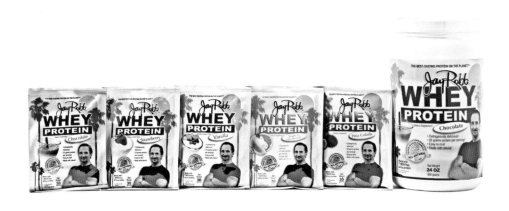

AGE LESS

1. Jay Robb Chocolate Whey Protein 30 grams: 0/0*
2. Jay Robb Strawberry Whey Protein 30 grams: 0/0*
3. Jay Robb Vanilla Whey Protein 30 grams: 0/0*
4. Jay Robb Tropical Dreamsicle Whey Protein 30 grams: 0/0*
5. Jay Robb Piña Colada Whey Protein 30 grams: 0/0*
6. Jay Robb Chocolate Whey Protein 24 oz: 0/0*

*contains stevia, an herbal sweetener that does not cause blood-sugar spikes

Chocolate

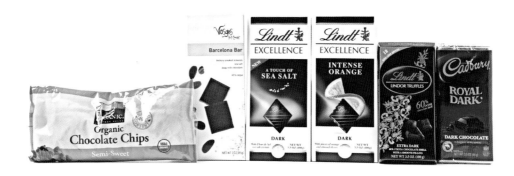

AGE MORE

1. 365 Everyday Value Organic Semi-Sweet Chocolate Chips: 8/1
2. Vosges Barcelona Bar 45% Cacao: 19/1
3. Lindt Excellence A Touch of Sea Salt Dark Chocolate: 19/2
4. Lindt Excellence Intense Orange Dark Chocolate: 17/2
5. Lindt Lindor Truffles Extra Dark 60% Cocoa Chocolate: 12/1
6. Cadbury Royal Dark Dark Chocolate: 20/2

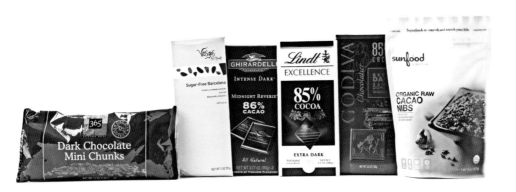

AGE LESS

1. 365 Everyday Value Dark Chocolate Mini Chunks: 4/1
2. Vosges Sugar-Free Barcelona: 3/1
3. Ghirardelli Intense Dark Midnight Reverie 86% Cacao: 5/1
4. Lindt Excellence 85% Cocoa Extra Dark: 5/1
5. Godiva 85% Cacao Extra Dark Santo Domingo Chocolate: 5/1
6. Sunfood Organic Raw Cacao Nibs: 0/1

Brownies & Cakes

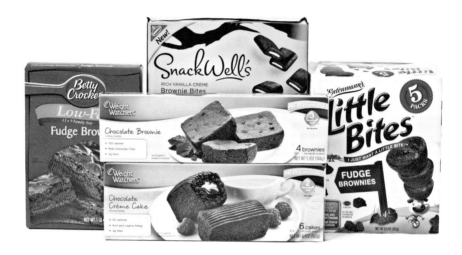

AGE MORE

1. Betty Crocker Low-Fat Fudge Brownie: 20/2
2. Weight Watchers Chocolate Crème Cake: 9/1
3. Weight Watchers Chocolate Brownies: 14/2
4. Entenmann's Fudge Brownies Little Bites: 17/2
5. SnackWell's Rich Vanilla Crème Brownie Bites: 13/2

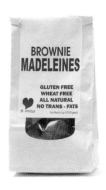
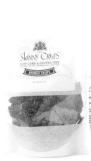
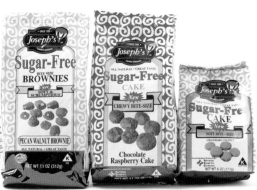

1. St. Amour Brownie Madeleines: 2/1
2. Skinny Crisps Brownie Crisps: 4/1
3. Joseph's Sugar-Free Pecan Walnut Bite Size Brownies: 0/1
4. Joseph's Sugar-Free Chocolate Raspberry Chewy Bite-Size Cake: 0/1
5. Joseph's Sugar-Free Strawberry Coconut Bite-Size Cake: 0/2

Chocolate Cookies

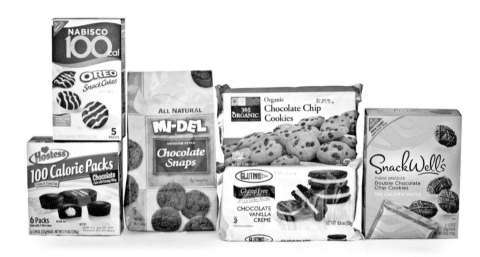

AGE MORE

1. Hostess Chocolate Cake with Creamy Filling 100 Calorie Packs: 11/2
2. Nabisco Oreo Snack Cakes 100 Cal: 9/1
3. Mi-Del Swedish Style Chocolate Snaps: 11/2
4. Glutino Chocolate Vanilla Crème Gluten Free Dream Cookies: 11/1
5. 365 Everyday Value Organic Chocolate Chip Cookies: 9/2
6. SnackWell's Fudge Drizzled Double Chocolate Chip Cookies 100 Calorie Packs: 7/1

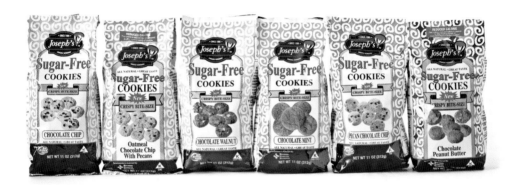

1. Joseph's Sugar-Free Chocolate Chip Cookies: 0/1
2. Joseph's Sugar-Free Oatmeal Chocolate Chip with Pecans Cookies: 0/1
3. Joseph's Sugar-Free Chocolate Walnut Cookies: 0/1
4. Joseph's Sugar-Free Chocolate Mint Cookies: 0/1
5. Joseph's Sugar-Free Pecan Chocolate Chip Cookies: 0/1
6. Joseph's Sugar-Free Chocolate Peanut Butter Cookies: 0/1

Chocolate Drinks

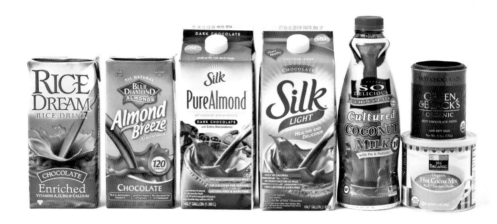

AGE MORE

1. Rice Dream Enriched Chocolate Rice Drink: 28/2
2. Blue Diamond Almond Breeze Chocolate Almond Milk: 20/2
3. Silk Pure Almond Dark Chocolate: 22/2
4. Silk Light Chocolate: 14/1
5. So Delicious Chocolate Cultured Coconut Milk: 19/2
6. 365 Everyday Value Organic Hot Cocoa Mix Rich Chocolate Flavor: 22/2
7. Green & Black's Organic Hot Chocolate Drink: 12/1

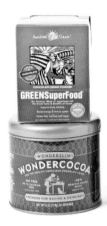
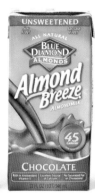
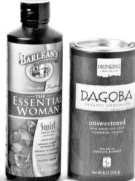

AGE LESS

1. Wonderslim Wondercocoa: 0/0
2. Blue Diamond Almond Breeze Unsweetened Chocolate Almond Milk: 0/0
3. Barlean's The Essential Woman Swirl: 0/1
4. Dagoba Unsweetened Organic Drinking Chocolate: 0/1
5. Amazing Grass Green SuperFood Chocolate Drink Powder: 0/0

6

Fat-Melting
Exercises

Weight-loss personalities have long championed exercise as the most effective way to feel young and drop unwanted inches from your waistline. Now that I've shared with you that hidden sugar is the *real* culprit when it comes to accelerated signs of aging and belly fat, it may seem strange that I would recommend exercise at all. The truth is, exercise is still incredibly valuable for overall health. By simply doing the exercises in this chapter for five minutes each morning, you will increase bone density, build muscle for a more shapely frame, and increase energy.

But first I need you to push aside all the images in your head of hard-bodied TV personalities yelling at sweaty clients on a treadmill or peddling some bizarre all-in-one contraption. Exercise alone will not produce the results you've been promised. I created the FAT-MELTING CARB SWAP™ to ensure that you can finally look and feel younger with a smaller waist for life. The simple exercise program in this chapter is designed as a supplement to The Aging Cure™ lifestyle, with some added benefits. Every routine in the next few pages has been created with you in mind, to ensure that it is fun, effective, and effortless.

As I've said over and over in this book, the true culprit of visible signs of aging and excess belly fat is hidden sugar.

Although cutting-edge science has revealed this truth for decades, there are still plenty of "powers that be" that continue to promote a different agenda. You've probably heard this familiar battle cry in the fight against obesity: "Eat less and exercise more." Now with the Aging Cure, you're learning about another strategy—one that really works—and it is this: to finally introduce the truth about hidden sugar and its impact on waistlines across the world.

That's why I was thrilled when a recent *Newsweek* article turned the spotlight on a fellow pioneer in the "sugar revolution," my friend Gary Taubes. Rarely will anyone in the "fight against obesity" challenge conventional wisdom to introduce the truth. But in this provocative article, Taubes opposed the conventional wisdom of some pretty heavy hitters with the revolutionary stance that is shared by The Aging Cure™: that calories carry little weight in the fight against obesity. I agree with him 100 percent. Of course, I also believe that exercise is still valuable for reasons separate from long-term weight loss.

Moderate exercise, such as the strength-training exercises in this chapter, has been proven to strengthen bone density. A recent study observed two separate groups of adults attempting to drop weight. One group modified their eating habits to promote a lower insulin load, the same way avoiding hidden sugar keeps that fat-controlling hormone balanced. The other group also modified their food intake, plus added light exercise. Both groups experienced lasting weight loss; however, the group that included moderate physical activity had a better bone density. Maintaining healthy bone density with five minutes of exercise each morning will assist in injury prevention and reduce your risk for osteoporosis, as well as helping you look and feel younger.

Bone density is becoming more of an issue for many of my clients who are concerned with aging. My good friend Dr. Christiane Northrup has been on the forefront of women's health for years and boasts a keen knowledge on how to age gracefully. One thing that both she and my clients are concerned about is osteoporosis.

As it turns out, strength training is not the only variable in keeping a healthy bone mass. When it comes to strong, healthy bones, Dr. Northrup and I both agree that it is also necessary to keep your glucose levels balanced by avoiding hidden sugar. High blood sugar results in an acidic pH in your body, which is detrimental to blood health. In an effort to bring balance to your pH level, the body pulls calcium from bones. When your diet is continually high in sugar, it decreases your bone mass and contributes to a common aging ailment: osteoporosis. By moderating your insulin with 15/6, you can significantly reduce the risk of weakening your bone structure.

Daily exercise is also a great way to give your body an energy boost. Moderate exercise promotes healthy circulation that energizes your system. Additionally, keeping your muscles active assists your body in burning its energy stores (fat, in other words). Mark Sisson describes it aptly when he says that walking "mobilizes some stored fats and gets the muscles burning them." As always, I do not suggest that you spend hours at the gym or on a treadmill while counting calories. That old conventional wisdom does not work long term. Moderating your insulin daily with my FAT-MELTING CARB SWAP™ is the true key to maintaining a healthy weight while looking and feeling youthful for life.

Move #1: Waist Whittler

On the floor, assume a push-up position. Slowly move your left knee to touch your left elbow, then return your knee to its original position and set your left foot to the floor. Repeat on the right side, moving your right knee to touch your right elbow. Alternate from right to left for 1 minute.

Modifications:

Easier: Standing up with your arms straight out in front of you, alternate lifting each leg, bending each knee so your knee is parallel with your hips.

Harder: Bring each knee to the opposite elbow to engage your obliques.

Move #2: Butt Buster

Lie with your back flat on the floor, with your arms flat by your sides and palms on the floor. Slide your feet so that they are a couple of inches in front of your knees. Raise your hips up off the floor, keeping your feet and arms flat on the floor. Squeeze your butt muscles as you raise your hips. Slowly return hips to the floor and repeat for 1 minute.

Modifications:

Easier: Take longer rests.

Harder: Keep your hips off the floor the entire time.

Move #3: Shoulder Shaper

Sit on the floor. With your knees bent, place your feet flat on the floor in front of you, a couple of inches in front of your knees. Place your hands several inches behind you with your palms flat on the floor, fingers facing forward. Slowly raise your hips up off the floor several inches, keeping feet and palms on the floor as you raise your hips. Dip your body down by bending your elbows. Continue to dip up and down, slowly returning to the floor, and repeat for 1 minute.

Modifications:

Easier: Assume the same position, but do not lift your hips off the floor. Continue to bend your elbows and dip your body up and down.

Harder: Sit on the edge of a sturdy chair and place your palms on the edge of the chair, fingers solidly gripping the chair. Move your legs out in front of you 6 inches past your knees. Feet should be flat on the floor. Move your buttocks forward and bend your elbows, and dip down and then back up.

Move #4: Chest Chiseler

Stand in front of a sturdy table an arm's length away. Reach your hands out directly in front of you and place your hands closer together so that your two index fingers and your two thumbs touch, forming a diamond shape with your hands. Make sure your thumbs are on the angle of the table to ensure you do not slide forward. Slowly bring your chest to your hands by bending your elbows, and then come back up. Repeat for 1 minute.

Modifications:

Easier: Stand an arm's length away from a sturdy wall, palms flat on the wall. Slowly bring your chest to your hands by bending your elbows, then push away again.

Harder: Assume a "modified" push-up position with your knees on the floor, feet lifted. Slowly lower yourself until you are a couple of inches off the floor, then push yourself back up.

Move #5: Thigh Trimmer

Stand with your feet hip-width apart. Raise your arms straight in front of you, palms facing downward, then bend your left knee and raise your left leg in front of you off of the floor about 6 inches. While keeping your knee bent and leg off the floor, slowly squat down by bending your right knee, maintaining your balance, keeping your arms raised; then return to standing. Repeat with right leg lifted off of the floor. Alternate from left to right for 1 minute.

Modifications:

Easier: Keep your left knee bent and lift your heel off the ground, while keeping your toes on the floor; slowly squat down, putting 80 percent of your weight on the right foot.

Harder: Instead of keeping your knee bent, keep the leg fully extended as you lift each foot off the ground in front of you.

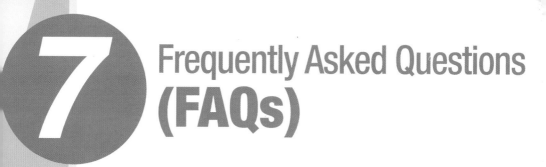

Frequently Asked Questions (FAQs)

1. Does sugar really age me?

Yes. Sugar ages you primarily through a process called *glycation,* in which sugar attaches to proteins (including the primary proteins responsible for smooth, wrinkle-free skin: collagen and elastin) and creates modified proteins called advanced glycation end products, or AGEs. Research published in *The Journal of Nutrition* recently confirmed the link between excess consumption of sugars and higher amounts of AGEs. As AGEs accumulate, your skin becomes dull, rigid, and prone to premature wrinkles. That means the sugar you consume each day will directly impact visible signs of aging, such as the lines on your face! By consuming only up to 15 grams of sugar a day, you will look and feel younger.

2. Is applying creams and lotions to my skin not enough?

The benefits of anti-aging creams are minimal. In truth, these products address the symptoms, not the disease. They may slightly improve skin quality but cannot address the aging that is happening *inside* of your body. Until you reduce glycation by bringing balance to your insulin levels and reducing your oxidative stress with anti-oxidant-rich meals, you will always be fighting an uphill battle against the visible signs of aging. The best alternative to anti-aging beauty products is my FAT-MELTING CARB SWAP™.

3. What is the FAT-MELTING CARB SWAP™?

If you're familiar with *The Belly Fat Cure*™, you know that the Carb Swap System is my trademarked eating method that guarantees you will automatically steer clear of foods full of the sweeteners and processed carbohydrates that keep insulin levels high and belly fat present. The secret to the Carb Swap System is that it ensures that you always hit my magical Sugar and Carb Value of 15/6.

The FAT-MELTING CARB SWAP™ automatically keeps you on track for 15/6 just like the original Carb Swap System, but it utilizes the power of antioxidants to restore vitality to your skin and health while still avoiding hidden sugar. By swapping high-sugar, Age More selections with low-sugar, antioxidant-rich alternatives, you will lose belly fat, feel younger, and reduce visible signs of aging.

4. Will including antioxidants in my diet actually combat aging?

You bet! My entire group of trusted health experts—Dr. Oz, Dr. Northrup, and Dr. Perricone—all agree that eating foods rich in antioxidants is absolutely essential for overall health and reducing visible signs of aging.

Antioxidants protect you from free-radical damage. Free radicals are unstable molecules that have lost one electron and are seeking a replacement. Antioxidants supply the extra electron that free radicals need before the free radicals grab it from susceptible tissue, like the collagen layer of your skin. These microscopic miracle workers help keep your skin free of wrinkles, balance your hormones, and prevent varicose veins. They are especially important because they aid in the prevention of disease, including cancer and coronary heart disease.

5. How can I incorporate more antioxidants into my daily diet?

Adding antioxidants to your food in small ways can have a great impact on overall health At lunch or dinner, it's easy to add some herbs or spices that are rich in anti-inflammatory antioxidants to your dish, such as parsley, mint, rosemary, thyme, and oregano. These will enhance flavor in addition to reducing the effects of aging. Snacking on seeds can also be an easy way to add antioxidants to your diet. A handful of pumpkin or sunflower seeds is a 0/0 snack!

The ORAC scale, as I mentioned in Chapter 2, is a good starting point in finding antioxidant-rich foods, but it's not the be-all and end-all. Be mindful of hidden sugar as you venture out on your own and explore new foods.

6. What exactly is a serving of carbohydrates?

One serving of carbohydrates is 5 to 20 grams; two servings is 21 to 40 grams; and three is 41 to 60 grams. You are allowed six servings of carbs throughout the day on *The Aging Cure*™. I strongly recommend you have three balanced meals, with no meal's S/C Value being greater than 5/2, and any snacks being a 0/0.

7. Can I have fewer than 15 grams of sugar and 6 servings of carbs?

Yes! Keep in mind that 15/6 is intended to be a maximum, not a target goal to reach. If you've reached a plateau or are looking to accelerate weight loss for an event, check out the Faster Results Menu on page 36.

8. Can I just stick to 120 grams of carbohydrates or less a day instead of tracking individual carb servings?

The short answer is no. Many clients want to eat tiny snacks throughout the day and "save" their sugar and carb allowance to binge on one big meal at night. Unfortunately, that large meal will send your insulin through the roof and lock in belly fat. In order to achieve and maintain balance with that fat-controlling hormone, it's best to track your servings and enjoy three meals of up to 5/2 throughout each day.

9. Why don't I track proteins and fats on this plan?

Fat and protein sources do not significantly drive up your insulin level, which is what triggers your body to hold on to fat, especially around your waistline. Studies done at Harvard University over the past decade have linked belly fat to sugar and processed carbohydrates—not fat or protein.

Protein and fat are processed by your body very differently than carbs are. However, that does *not* mean you can eat a whole cow or ten sticks of butter! You should only continue to eat if you still feel hungry. The good news is that protein and fat sources satiate your hunger quickly, so you're less likely to overeat.

10. Should I be worried about my cholesterol levels increasing on this program?

If you have high cholesterol, I recommend speaking with your doctor before starting any weight-loss plan. However, it's more likely that *The Aging Cure*™ will help decrease your cholesterol levels rather than raise them. In fact, some studies reveal sugar to be the largest contributor to high cholesterol. Many sugars travel directly to your liver and get converted to fat, which is sent into your blood, increasing your LDL levels (otherwise known as bad cholesterol).

11. Why do I count the sugar and carbs in fruit and vegetables? I thought they were healthy!

If your goal is truly to get rid of belly fat, then you have to stick to no more than 15 grams of sugar and 6 servings of carbs each day, from *all* food sources. Fructose, the sugar found in fruit, has specifically been linked to belly fat—since it goes directly to the liver to be processed, it gets converted to fat and leads to visceral belly fat and high cholesterol. Keep in mind that throughout history, fruit was available only during

certain times of the year. Now we have access to fruit year-round in unlimited quanti-
ties, which is not how we were intended to consume it. Even though vegetables contain
many nutrients, they're still carbohydrates that get converted to glucose and so must
be counted for belly-fat loss.

12. Why is the S/C Value the same for different body sizes?

The S/C Value is designed to make sure that your body is keeping insulin low and
producing the appetite-suppressing hormone leptin—no matter what your gender, age,
or size—while also ensuring that you get enough servings of complex carbs a day. If you
have a larger body type and feel that you need more food, you can try eating more protein, fats, or some of the lower-sugar vegetables (mostly the green ones!). The goal is to
follow the S/C Value and eat until you're satisfied within those requirements.

13. Where can I look up the S/C Values of foods?

Throughout this book, you'll find the S/C Value of all meals and food products pictured.
You can also turn to my newly updated *Belly Fat Cure™ Sugar & Carb Counter,* which includes
thousands of other food items (including restaurant foods!) listed with their S/C Value.

14. Should I still keep track of how many calories I'm eating?

Counting calories is not the most effective way to moderate your eating and drop belly fat. I strongly believe that it is not how many calories you are eating that counts; it's the
type of calories. Monitoring your consumption of sugars and carbs—the only foods that
significantly impact insulin production—is the key to weight loss. Simply apply the S/C
Value to your daily eating, and you'll be successful in your weight loss and maintenance.

15. Why must I avoid synthetic sugars (aspartame, sucralose, and saccharin)?

These substances are known as *excitotoxins*. This means that they "overexcite" neurons in the brain, causing degeneration and even death in important nerve cells. When too many nerve cells die, your nervous system begins to malfunction, and it can't communicate with other parts of your body. This can ultimately lead to nervous-system disorders such as Parkinson's disease, multiple sclerosis, and Alzheimer's disease.

16. What are sugar alcohols, and do I have to count them?

Sugar alcohols don't actually contain any sugar or alcohol. They're a type of carbohydrate that requires little insulin to be converted to energy. They are used in foods for sweetness, but don't cause a significant spike in blood sugar or inhibit your immune system in any way. On *The Aging Cure*™, you do not need to count any grams listed as "sugar alcohols" in the sugar category; they may, however, be counted on a label under "total carbohydrates," which means that they will be included as carbs in the S/C Value (but you won't have to track them separately).

Be aware that tolerance for sugar alcohols can vary from person to person. Moderate consumption of any sugar alcohol should cause no digestive issues, but excess consumption can lead to gas and bloating, so do pay attention to your own personal level of tolerance. Research has shown that erythritol is the least likely to cause intestinal distress because it is almost completely absorbed by your small intestines and excreted in urine.

17. Can I eat as many 0/0 items as I want, or is there a limit?

If a food has absolutely no sugar or carb grams, you can enjoy more than one serving. Green tea is one of the few items of which you can have an unlimited amount.

Some 0/0 items contain carbs but remain under 5 grams for one serving only. For example, one packet of Truvia—a recommended sweetener on *The Aging Cure*™—contains

3 grams of carbs per serving. Consuming two packets of Truvia, however, brings your carb gram total to 6, which must then be counted as one serving for your day.

18. I'm a vegetarian and my partner is vegan . . . can we do this program?

Yes. Although I believe that animals are the best source of protein, you both can simply substitute the meats and/or cheeses I recommend in this program for your favorite vegan or vegetarian options. Just be sure that you know the sugar and carbohydrate content of these substitutes. (Please also refer to my Vegan/Vegetarian menu on page 44.)

19. Can I do this program if I'm following a gluten-free diet?

Yes. Since the program is based on a simple, clean way of eating, it can easily be adapted to be gluten-free.

20. Can I do this program if I'm pregnant?

If you are pregnant or are breast-feeding, please check with your doctor before beginning *The Aging Cure*™.

21. Can I still do this program if I'm training for a half marathon, marathon, or triathlon?

A common misconception is that runners or endurance athletes need lots of complex carbs for energy. However, when you're not providing your body with a constant stream of carbs to burn, your body naturally taps into your fat stores for energy. Even runners and endurance athletes will do their bodies a favor by switching to a fat-burning metabolism instead of a carb-burning (and fat-storing) metabolism.

22. If I have an allergy to one of the Age Less foods, can I still do this program?

You can absolutely still succeed on this program if you are allergic to nuts, dairy, eggs, and so on. Simply substitute another like food for the one to which you are allergic. For example, if you are allergic to nuts, choose another Age Less snack instead, like cheese or deli meat.

23. Can my kids eat this way?

Definitely! Limiting sugar in your children's diet and replacing it with smarter options will increase overall health. Low-sugar, nutrient-rich foods are equally beneficial for your kids as they are for you. It may be difficult to change your kids' minds about sugar if they have fallen into a habit of constantly eating sugary snacks, but please do not let this discourage you from guiding them to a healthier lifestyle.

I suggest you lead by example first. Then get your children involved by teaching them about the benefits of certain foods and letting them help you prepare snacks and meals. Your kids will be more interested in the foods they're eating if they help create the meals with you. Try to make cooking something fun that your entire family can enjoy together.

24. Why am I not losing weight?

If you notice that your waistline isn't decreasing, or it's even increasing, be sure you're sticking to 15/6. However, it's more likely that what you're measuring is actually "false" belly fat. If you add more fiber to your diet than you're used to and aren't hydrated enough, you can accumulate false belly fat due to waste buildup.

If you're drinking plenty of water and your elimination is still sluggish, your gut bacteria may be low (this is especially true if you've been taking antibiotics). The bacteria in your gut aid in *peristalsis,* the rhythmic contraction of the intestinal walls that literally keeps things moving. By simply adding a probiotic supplement to your diet, you can restore a healthy balance of beneficial bacteria that will make it easier for your body to clear the waste more efficiently. Also, be sure to get dietary fiber from other food sources such as brown rice, whole-wheat breads, and vegetables like artichokes and broccoli.

25. Do I need to incorporate probiotics into *The Aging Cure*™?

Constipation is the biggest reason people fail on low-carb diets, and probiotics are very helpful with this condition. Although they are not essential, I would recommend that you begin this program with probiotics to ensure a smooth transition. If at any time you fail to have a bowel movement for 48 hours, definitely begin incorporating probiotics.

26. I'm taking probiotics, but things still aren't moving . . . help!

I recommend eating more vegetables that are high in fiber, such as broccoli and artichokes. If things are still sluggish after incorporating probiotics and more veggies into your diet, I suggest adding one or two servings of a soluble fiber supplement.

27. What do I do if I hit a plateau?

Many of my clients find the Faster Results Menu (on page 36) to be very helpful in breaking through plateaus. Alternatively, consider that there might be something that is stimulating insulin in your food. Be sure to check all dressings, sauces, and drinks you're consuming for sugar or artificial sweeteners. Get back to basics and be diligent about tracking what you eat. If you hit a plateau, chances are you may not be sticking to 15/6. Tracking what you eat each day will help you stay accountable and make sure that you're eating exactly what you need to maximize belly fat loss.

Also, I recommend that you pay attention to how much fiber you're getting each day—aim for 25 to 30 grams, and you'll be amazed by how quickly your belly fat disappears. Finally, keep in mind that as you near your goal weight, your weight loss will naturally slow down a bit.

28. Do I need to exercise to lose belly fat?

No. Many of my clients have lost weight just by changing the way they eat. However, once they lost their belly fat, many of them felt so good that they added exercise in. While it isn't crucial to exercise to lose belly fat, I believe that exercise is still part of a healthy lifestyle. You don't have to spend hours on the treadmill each day, though! Even just power walking for 20 minutes each morning can be greatly beneficial.

29. Can I drink alcohol on this program?

Yes, you can enjoy alcohol in moderation. I suggest a glass of red wine in the evening with dinner, which has the added benefit of antioxidants. However, if you find that you're not losing weight on this program, I recommend avoiding alcohol.

30. What if I can't find the specific products mentioned in the book?

Most of the products mentioned in this book can be purchased online if you're unable to find them in stores; however, it is not necessary to buy any specialty items in order to have success on this program. All you truly need—protein and vegetables—can be found in any grocery store nationwide.

31. How do I correctly measure my waist?

First, suck in your belly as tight as you can. Next, measure your waist around your belly button with a tape measure. (To view a video demonstration of Dr. Oz and me measuring our waists, visit JorgeCruise.com.)

32. Where can I share my weight-loss success?

Share your story—with before-and-after photos!—on my Facebook page: Facebook.com/JorgeCruiseFan.

33. Where can I connect with you further?

If you'd like to receive even more recipes and menus, visit JorgeCruise.com. There you'll find an array of free tools and keep updated with new coaching programs, events, and the latest interviews on healthy eating.

Index of Meals

BEEF & PORK

Garlic-Grilled Rib Eye 117

Juicy Ham and Tomato Sandwich 73

Robust Roast Beef Wrap 93

Savory Roast Beef and Swiss Melt 75

Sweet and Tangy Ham-Salad Pita 97

Tangy Roast Beef Wrap. 91

BURGERS

Creamy Crab Sliders 69

Garlic-Spinach Turkey Burger. 67

EGG DISHES

Creamy Egg-Salad Wraps with Spicy Popcorn . . . 87

Goat Cheese and Zucchini Frittata 51

Sharp Cheddar Ham Frittata. 49

FISH & SEAFOOD DISHES

Creamy Tuna Wrap 85

Crème Fraîche and Salmon Sandwich. 71

Crispy Crab Curry 77

Garlic and Saffron Mussels. 123

Parmesan Dill Halibut 119

Parmesan Tilapia with Mint Risotto 121

MEATLESS DISHES

Apple and Olive Wrap 89

Savory Curry Chickpea Pita 99

Sizzling Spinach-Mushroom Quesadilla 103

Spicy Tofu Tacos 101

PASTA

Pancetta Penne 63

Zesty Chicken Bacon Linguine. 65

PIZZA

Artichoke, Onion, and Olive Pizza 57

Cheesy Pizza Strips. 61

Cheesy Supreme Pizza 53

Perfect Margherita Pizza. 55

Sweet and Savory Gorgonzola Pizza. 59

POULTRY DISHES

Chicken and Broccoli Stir Fry 109

Creamy Caesar Turkey Wrap 81

Creamy Goat-Cheese Stuffed Chicken 115

Crispy Chicken Parmesan. 105

Crispy Chicken Strips 111

Savory Sage Chicken Marsala 107

Spicy Chicken Kebabs 113

Sweet Curry Turkey Pita 95

Turkey and Salsa Wrap 83

Zesty Pesto Turkey with Parmesan Popcorn. 79

SALADS

Crunchy Carrot and Cashew Salad 147

Crunchy Salmon Salad 141

Fresh and Spicy Garden Salad. 133

Goat Cheese and Shrimp Salad. 139

Juicy Pear and Pecan Salad. 145

Lemon-Spiced Shrimp Salad 137

Prosciutto and Goat Cheese Salad 129

Ranch BBQ Chopped Salad. 127

Rich Roast Beef and Hazelnut Salad. 131

Salmon and Sourdough Salad 143

Summer Blueberry Chicken Salad. 125

Tangy Greek Arugula Salad 135

Tangy Sesame Sourdough Chicken Salad 149

TREATS

Creamy Peanut Butter–Covered Strawberries . . . 153

Sweet Lemonade Dream Bars 155

Sweet Vanilla Cream Bourbon 157

Vanilla, Pecan, and Espresso Sundae 151

Bibliography

CHAPTER 1

"Abdominal fat and what to do about it." *Harvard Women's Health Watch.* December 2006.
http://www.health.harvard.edu/newsweek/Abdominal-fat-and-what-to-do-about-it.html.

Barclay L. "Waist Girth Predicts Cardiovascular Risk Better Than BMI." *Medscape Medical News.*
September 23, 2002.

Barzilai, N, G Gupta. "Interaction between aging and syndrome X: new insights on the pathophysiology of
fat distribution." *Annals of the New York Academy of Sciences.* 892 (1999):58–72.

Behan KJ, J Mbizo. "The relationship between waist circumference and biomarkers for diabetes and CVD
in healthy non-obese women." *Laboratory Medicine.* 38 (2007):422–427.

Buss, D. "Strategies of Human Mating." *Psychological Topics.* 15 (2006):239–260

Demetra DC, PP Jones, AE Pimentel, et al. "Increased abdominal-to-peripheral fat distribution contributes
to altered autonomic-circulatory control with human aging." *The American Journal of Physiology—Heart
and Circulatory Physiology.* 287 (2004):H1530–H1537.

Despres, JP, S Moorjani, PJ Lupien, et al. "Regional distribution of body fat, plasma lipoproteins, and
cardiovascular disease." *Arteriosclerosis, Thrombosis, and Vascular Biology.* 10 (1990):497–511.

Fisher ML, M Voracek. "The shape of beauty: determinants of female physical attractiveness." *Journal of
Cosmetic Dermatology.* 5 (2006):190–4.

Fontana L, JC Eagon, ME Trujillo, et al. "Visceral Fat Adipokine Secretion Is Associated with Systemic
Inflammation in Obese Humans." *Diabetes.* 56 (2007):1010–1013.

Forouhi, NG, N Sattar, PM McKeigue. "Relation of C-reactive protein to body fat distribution and features
of the metabolic syndrome in Europeans and South Asians." *International Journal of Obesity and Related
Metabolic Disorders.* 25 (2001):1327–31.

Higginbotham, S, ZF Zhang, IM Lee, et al. "Dietary Glycemic Load and Risk of Colorectal Cancer in the
Women's Health Study." *Journal of the National Cancer Institute.* 96 (2004):229–233.

Janssen, I, PT Katzmarzyk, R Ross. "Waist circumference and not body mass index explains obesity-
related health risk." *American Journal of Clinical Nutrition.* 79 (2004):379–384.

Larsson, SC, L Bergkvist, A Wolk. "Consumption of sugar and sugar-sweetened foods and the risk of
pancreatic cancer in a prospective study." *American Journal of Clinical Nutrition.* 84 (2006):1171–1176.

Liese, AD, M Schulz, F Fang, et al. "Dietary Glycemic Index and Glycemic Load, Carbohydrate and Fiber Intake, and Measures of Insulin Sensitivity, Secretion, and Adiposity in the Insulin Resistance Atherosclerosis Study." *Diabetes Care.* 28 (2005):2832–2838.

Mayo Clinic Staff. "Belly Fat in Women: How to Keep it Off." April 2007. http://www.mayoclinic.com/health/belly-fat/WO00128

Passmore, R, YE Swindells. "Observations on the respiratory quotients and weight gain of man after eating large quantity of carbohydrate." *British Journal of Nutrition.* 17 (163):331–339.

Pischon T, H Boeing, K Hoffman, et al. "General and Abdominal Adiposity and Risk of Death in Europe." *The New England Journal of Medicine.* 359 (2008):2105–2120.

Resnick, HE, EA Carter, M Aloia, et al. "Cross-sectional relationship of reported fatigue to obesity, diet, and physical activity: results from the third national health and nutrition examination survey." *Journal of Clinical Sleep Medicine.* 2 (2006):163–9.

Sanchez, A, Reeser, JL, Lau, HS, et al. "Role of sugars in human neutrophilic phagocytosis." *American Journal of Clinical Nutrition.* 26 (1973):1180–1184.

Singh, D. "Adaptive Significance of Female Physical Attractiveness: Role of Waist-to-Hip Ratio." *Journal of Personality and Social Psychology.* 65 (1993):293–307.

———. "Waist-to-hip ratio and judgment of attractiveness and healthiness of female figures by male and female physicians." *International Journal of Obesity and Related Metabolic Disorders.* 18 (1994):731–7.

Streeter SA, DH McBurney. "Waist-hip ratio and attractiveness. New evidence and a critique of 'a critical test.'" *Evolution and Human Behavior.* 24 (2003):88–98.

Tavani, A, L Giordano, S Gallus, et al. C. "Consumption of sweet foods and breast cancer risk in Italy." *Annals of Oncology.* 17 (2006):341–345.

Vatanparast, H, PD Chilibeck, SM Cornish, et al. "DXA-derived Abdominal Fat Mass, Waist Circumference, and Blood Lipids in Postmenopausal Women." *Obesity.* (2009).

Yalow, RS, SA Berson. "Immunoassay of Endogenous Plasma Insulin in Man." *Journal of Clinical Investigation.* 39 (1960):1157–75.

Yalow, RS, SM Glick, J Roth, et. al. "Plasma Insulin and Growth Hormone Levels in Obesity and Diabetes." *Annals of the New York Academy of Sciences.* 131 (1965):357–73.

Zhang C, KM Rexrode, RM van Dam, et al. "Abdominal obesity and the risk of all-cause, cardiovascular, and cancer mortality: sixteen years of follow-up in US women." *Circulation.* 117 (2008):1658–67.

CHAPTER 2

B. Conti, "Considerations on Temperature, Longevity and Aging," *Cellular and Molecular Life Sciences.* 65, no. 11 (June 2008).

Baldauf, Sarah. "Too Fat? No More Excuses." *U.S. News Health.* 31 December 2007.

Basciano H, L Federico, K Adeli, et al. "Fructose, insulin resistance, and metabolic dyslipidemia." *Nutrition & Metabolism.* 2 (2005):5.

Beltramo E, Berrone E, Buttiglieri S, Porta M. "Thiamine and benfotiamine prevent increased apoptosis in endothelial cells and pericytes cultured in high glucose." *Diabetes Metab Res Rev.* 2004 Jul–Aug;20(4):330-6.

Beltramo E, Berrone E, Tarallo S, Porta M. "Different apoptotic responses of human and bovine pericytes to fluctuating glucose levels and protective role of thiamine." *Diabetes Metab Res Rev.* 2009 Sep;25(6):566-76.

Bergman RN, SP Kim, IR Hsu, et al. "Abdominal Obesity: Role in the Pathophysiology of Metabolic Disease and Cardiovascular Risk." *American Journal of Medicine.* 120 (2007):S3–S8.

Beyer, PL, EM Caviar, and RW McCallum. "Fructose Intake at Current Levels in the United States May Cause Gastrointestinal Distress in Normal Adults." *Journal of the American Dietetic Association.* 105 (2005):1559–66.

"BUSM Researchers Identify Key Regulator of Inflammatory Response." HealthCanal.com. http://www.healthcanal.com/immune-system/28425-BUSM-Researchers-Identify-Key-Regulator-Inflammatory-Response.html

"Can Food Forestall Aging?" *Agricultural Research.* Feb. 1999. 14–17.

Cleave, TL. *The Saccharine Disease.* New Canaan, CT: Keats Publishing, August 1975.

Cohen, PG. "Obesity in men: The hypogonadal-estrogen receptor relationship and its effect on glucose homeostasis." *Medical Hypotheses.* 70 (2008):358–360.

Cordain L, SB Eaton, A Sebastian, et al. "Origins and evolution of the Western diet: health implications for the 21st century." *American Journal of Clinical Nutrition.* 81 (2005):341–354.

Delaney, Brian M.; Walford, Lisa (2010-05-25). *The Longevity Diet: The Only Proven Way to Slow the Aging Process and Maintain Peak Vitality—Through Calorie Restriction* (Kindle Locations 4479–4480). Perseus Books Group. Kindle Edition.

E. J. Masoro, "Antiaging Action of Caloric Restriction: Endocrine and Metabolic Aspects," *Obesity Research* 3, suppl. 2 (September 1995).

Fung, TT, V Malik, KM Rexrode, et al. "Sweetened beverage consumption and risk of coronary heart disease in women." *American Journal of Clinical Nutrition.* 89 (2009):1037–1042.

Gordon, ES, M Goldgerg, GJ Chosy. "A New Concept in the Treatment of Obesity." *The Journal of the American Medical Association.* 186 (1963):50–60.

Hesketh, K, E Waters, J Green, et al. "Healthy Eating, activity and obesity prevention: a qualitative study of parent and child perceptions in Australia." *Health Promotion International.* 20 (2005):19–26.

McGlothin, P, Averill M. *The CR Way: Using the Secrets of Calorie Restriction for a Longer, Healthier Life.* NY: HarperCollins; 2008:57–78

Newsholme, EA, C Start. *Regulation in Metabolism.* New York: John Wiley, 1973.

N. Pitsikas, M. Carli, S. Fidecka, and S. Algeri, "Effect of Life-long Hypocaloric Diet on Age-Related Changes in Motor and Cognitive Behavior in a Rat Population," *Neurobiology of Aging.* 11, no. 4 (July–Aug 1990).

Ohio State University Center for Clinical and Translational Science. "Does Fatty Food Impact Marital Stress?" *Newswise.* http://www.healthcanal.com/immune-system/28425-BUSM-Researchers-Identify-Key-Regulator-Inflammatory-Response.html

R. Weindruch, "Caloric Restriction and Aging," *Scientific American.* 274, no. 1 (January 1996): 46–52.

Schulze, MB, JE Manson, D S Ludwig, et al. "Sugar-Sweetened Beverages, Weight Gain, and Incidence of Type 2 Diabetes in Young and Middle-Aged Women." *The Journal of the American Medical Association.* 292 (2004):927–934.

Stanhope, K, P Havel. "Fructose Consumption: Considerations for Future Research on Its Effects on Adipose Distribution, Lipid Metabolism, and Insulin Sensitivity in Humans." *The Journal of Nutrition.* 139 (2009):1236S–1241S.

Stanhope, KL, PJ Havel. "Fructose Consumption: Potential Mechanisms for its Effects to Increase Visceral Adiposity and Induce Dyslipidemia and Insulin Resistance." *Current Opinion in Lipidology.* 19 (2008):16–24.

Stirban A, Negrean M, Stratmann B, et al. "Benfotiamine prevents macro- and microvascular endothelial dysfunction and oxidative stress following a meal rich in advanced glycation end products in individuals with type 2 diabetes." *Diabetes Care.* 2006 Sep;29(9):2064–71.

Teff, KL, SS Elliott, M Tschop, et al. "Dietary Fructose Reduces Circulating Insulin and Leptin, Attenuates Postprandial Suppression of Ghrelin, and Increases Triglycerides in Women." *The Journal of Clinical Endocrinology & Metabolism.* 89 (2004):2963–2972.

Vlassara H, Palace MR. Glycoxidation: the menace of diabetes and aging. *Mt Sinai J Med.* 2003 Sep;70(4):232–41.

Woodham, Chai. "You May Be Fat and Not Even Know it." *U.S. News Health.* 30 April 2012.

CHAPTER 3

Abou-Donia, MB, EM El-Masry, AA Abdel-Rahman, et al. "Splenda Alters Gut Microflora and Increases Intestinal P-Glycoprotein and Cytochrome P-450 in Male Rats." *Journal of Toxicology and Environmental Health.* Part A 71 (2008):1415–1429.

Arrigoni, E, F Brouns, R Amado. "Human gut microbiota does not ferment erythritol." *British Journal of Nutrition.* 94 (2005):643–646.

Batterham, M, R Cavanagh, A Jenkins, et al. "High-protein meals may benefit fat oxidation and energy expenditure in individuals with higher body fat." *Nutrition & Dietetics.* 65 (2008):246–252.

Krajcovicová-Kudláčková, M, Kebeková, R Schinzel, et al. "Advanced Glycation End Products and Nutrition." *Physiology Research.* 51 (2002):313–316.

Levi, B, MJ Werman. "Long-term fructose consumption accelerates glycation and several age-related variables in male rats." *The Journal of Nutrition.* 128 (1998):1442–9.

Maher, TJ, RJ Wurtmant. "Possible Neurologic Effects of Aspartame, a Widely Used Food Additive." *Environmental Health Perspectives.* 75 (1987):53–57.

Olney JW, NB Farber, E Spitznagel, et al. "Increasing brain tumor rates: is there a link to aspartame?" *Journal of Neuropathology and Experimental Neurology.* 55 (1996):1115–23.

Savita, SM, K Sheela, S Sunanda, et al. "Health Implications of Stevia Rebaudiana." *Journal of Human Ecology.* 15 (2004):191–194.

Vgontzas, AN, DA Papanicolaou, EO Bixler, et al. "Sleep Apnea and Daytime Sleepiness and Fatigue: Relation to Visceral Obesity, Insulin Resistance, and Hypercytokinemia." *The Journal of Clinical Endocrinology & Metabolism.* 85 (2000):1151–1158.

Walton RG, Hudak R, Green-Waite RJ. "Adverse reactions to aspartame: double-blind challenge in patients from a vulnerable population." *Biological Psychiatry.* 34 (1993):13–7.

CHAPTER 6

Cloud, John. "Why Exercise Won't Make You Thin." *Time.* 17 Aug. 2009: 42–47.

DeBusk, R. F., et al. "Training effects of long versus short bouts of exercise in healthy subjects." *The American Journal of Cardiology.* 65.15 (1990): 1010–3.

Evans, William J., and Joseph G. Cannon. "The Metabolic Effects of Exercise-Induced Muscle Damage." *Exercise and Sport Sciences Reviews.* 19.1 (1991): 99–126.

Lemon, Peter W. R. "Effects of Exercise on Protein Requirements." *Journal of Sports Sciences.* 9.S1 (1991): 53–70.

McArdle, William D., Frank I. Katch, and Victor L. Katch. *Exercise Physiology: Energy, Nutrition, and Human Performance.* Philadelphia: Lippincott Williams & Wilkins, 2007.

National Center for Health Statistics. "Prevalence of overweight, obesity and extreme obesity among adults: United States, trends 1960–62 through 2005–2006." Centers for Disease Control and Prevention. http://cdc.gov/nchs/data/hestat/overweight/overweight_adult.htm.

Tipton, Charles M. *American College of Sports Medicine's Advanced Exercise Physiology.* Philadelphia: Lippincott Williams & Wilkins, 2006.

Tjonna, Arnt Erik, et al. "Aerobic Interval Training Versus Continuous Moderate Exercise as a Treatment for the Metabolic Syndrome: A Pilot Study." *Circulation.* 118 (2008): 346–54.

Urhausen, A., H. Gabriel, and W. Kindermann. "Blood hormones as markers of training stress and overtraining." *Sports Medicine.* 20.4 (1995), 251–76.

Verger, P., M. T. Lanteaume, and J. Louis-Sylvestre. "Human intake and choice of foods at intervals after exercise." *Appetite.* 18.2 (1992): 93–99.

Warburton, Darren, Crystal Whitney Nicol, and Shannon Bredin. "Health benefits of physical activity: the evidence." *The Canadian Medical Association Journal.* 174.6 (2006): 801–9.

ADDITIONAL SOURCES

Barzilai, N, J Wang, D Massilon, et al. "Leptin Selectively Decreases Visceral Adiposity and Enhances Insulin Action." *The Journal of Clinical Investigation.* 100 (1997):3105–3110.

Chan P, X Dy, JC Liu, et al. "The effect of stevioside on blood pressure and plasma catecholamines in spontaneously hypertensive rats." *Life Sciences.* 63 (1998):1679–84.

Clapp, R, D Davis, S Epstein, et al. "National Toxicology Program Board of Scientific Counselors' Report on Carcinogens Subcommittee." *CSPI Reports.* October 24, 1997.

Costello, D. "The Price of Obesity." *Los Angeles Times.* April 1, 2005.

Diamant M, JL Hildo, MA van de Ree, et al. "The Association between Abdominal Visceral Fat and Carotid Stiffness Is Mediated by Circulating Inflammatory Markers in Uncomplicated Type 2 Diabetes." *The Journal of Clinical Endocrinology & Metabolism.* 90 (2005):1495–1501.

Ellwood M. "Fall's Fashion Makes the Waist More Important Than Ever." *New York Daily News.* October 4, 2007.

Deardorff, J. "Agave provokes a bitter debate as a sweetener." *Chicago Tribune.* March 23, 2008.

Falta, W. *Endocrine Diseases, Including Their Diagnosis and Treatment.* Philadelphia: P. Blakiston's Son & Co. 1923.

Gosnell M. "Killer Fat." *Discover.* February 2007.

Katcher, HI, RS Legro, AR Kunselman, et al. "The Effects of a Whole Grain-Enriched Hypocaloric Diet on Cardiovascular Disease Risk Factors in Men and Women With Metabolic Syndrome." *American Journal of Clinical Nutrition.* 87 (2008):79–90.

Liu G, CL Hughes, R Mathur, et al. "Metabolic effects of dietary lactose in adult female rats." *Reproduction Nutrition Development.* 2003 Nov–Dec;43 (6):567–76.

Mulligan, K, K Hootan, JM Schwarz, et al. "The Effects of Recombinant Human Leptin on Visceral Fat, Dyslipidemia, and Insulin Resistance in Patients with Human Immunodeficiency Virus-Associated Lipoatrophy and Hypoleptinemia." *Journal of Clinical Endocrinology & Metabolism.* 94 (2009):1137–1144.

Öhman MK, Y Shen, CI Obimba, et al. "Visceral Adipose Tissue Inflammation Accelerates Atherosclerosis in Apolipoprotein E–Deficient Mice." *Circulation.* 117 (2008):798–805.

Pagan, JA. and A Davila. "Obesity, Occupational Attainment, and Earnings." *Social Science Quarterly.* 78 (1997):756–70.

Pasquali, R. "Obesity, fat distribution and infertility." *Maturitas.* 54 (2006):363–371.

Price, GM, CG Biava, BL Oser, et al. "Bladder Tumors in Rats Fed Cyclohexylamine or High Doses of a Mixture of Cyclamate and Saccharin." *Science.* 167 (1970):1131–1132.

Reitzes, D. "Self and Health: Factors Influencing Self-Esteem and Functional Health." Paper presented at the annual meeting of the American Sociological Association, Marriott Hotel, Loews Philadelphia Hotel, Philadelphia, PA, Aug 12, 2005.

Rosch PJ. "All Obesity Is Not Created Equal." *Science.* 301 (2003):1325.

Sanches FMR, CM Avesani, MA Kamimura, et al. "Waist Circumference and Visceral Fat in CKD: A Cross-sectional Study." *American Journal of Kidney Diseases.* 52 (2008):66–73

Sztanke K, Pasternak K. "The Maillard Reaction and Its Consequences for a Living Body." *Ann Univ Mariae Curie Sklodowska Med.* 2003;58(2):159-62

Tilg H, AR Moschen. "Adipocytokines: mediators linking adipose tissue, inflammation and immunity." *Nature Reviews Immunology.* 6 (2006)772–783.

Tracy RP. "Is Visceral Adiposity the 'Enemy Within'?" *Arteriosclerosis, Thrombosis, and Vascular Biology.* 21 (2001):881–883.

Wang Y, MA Beydoun, L Liang, et al. "Will all Americans become overweight or obese? Estimating the progression and cost of the US obesity epidemic." *Obesity.* 16 (2008):2323–30.

Wass P, U Waldenstrom, S Rossner, et al. "An android body fat distribution in females impairs the pregnancy rate of in-vitro fertilization-embryo transfer." *Human Reproduction.* 12 (1997):2057–2060.

Whitaker, RC, JA Wright, MS Pepe, et al. "Predicting Obesity in Young Adulthood from Childhood and Parental Obesity." *The New England Journal of Medicine.* 337 (1997):869–873.

Zagorsky, JL. "Health and Wealth: The Late-20th Century Obesity Epidemic in the U.S." *Economics & Human Biology.* 3 (2005):296–313.

Acknowledgments

No book is ever completed without the support of a great team.

To the wonderful Hay House team—the sublime and youthful Louise Hay; Reid Tracy, Shannon Littrell, Charles McStravick, Christy Salinas, Johanne Mahaffey, John Thompson, and Lindsay McGinty; and, most especially, Stacey Smith—thank you for making this project an amazing experience.

To Kristin Penne, for keeping us all organized, on time, and sane. To Oliver Stephenson, for your ability to style food beautifully and the complete execution of this book; I couldn't do it without you. Thank you to Jared Davis for the cover photo. Thank you to Evan Dollard for the life and energy you gave to the written word, as well as your beautiful photography of the meals. To Blair Atkins, for your ability to research and dig up the hidden truths that built this book. To Paige Hill, for all your support with this project. To Michelle McGowen, for being a true asset. All of you make up my core team, and your hard work and incredible talents are invaluable. I can't thank you all enough for your dedication and commitment to creating outstanding content.

A very special thank-you to my invaluable circle of experts: Gary Taubes, Dr. Robert Lustig, Dr. Mehmet Oz, and Michael Pollan.

To my clients—your support in helping me refine this program, offering your comments, tips, and the courage to change your own lives, has been a gift. Thank you.

Thank you also to Rachael Ray, Kelly Ripa, Katie Couric, Al Roker, Diane Sawyer, Robin Roberts, Suze Orman, Pennie Clark Ianniciello, Ginnie Roeglin, Richard Gilante, Dr. Christiane Northrup, all my friends at **HayHouseRadio.com**, all the ladies on *The View,* and all my friends at *Extra* TV. And, of course, to Oprah Winfrey, for believing in me and helping me launch my career over a decade ago.

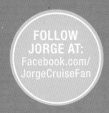

About the Author

JORGE CRUISE used to be 40 pounds overweight. Today, he is internationally recognized as America's #1 easy-diet expert and is the author of six consecutive *New York Times* best-selling series, with more than six million books in print in over 15 languages, including *The Belly Fat Cure, 8 Minutes in the Morning, The 3-Hour Diet, The 12-Second Sequence,* and *Body at Home.* He is also a contributing editor for *The Costco Connection* magazine, *First for Women* magazine, *Women's World* magazine, and *Extra* TV. He has appeared on *The Oprah Winfrey Show, The Dr. Oz Show,* CNN, *Good Morning America,* the *Today* show, *The Rachael Ray Show, Dateline NBC,* and *The View.*

Jorge received his bachelor's degree from the University of California, San Diego (UCSD); and has fitness credentials from the Cooper Institute for Aerobics Research, the American College of Sports Medicine (ACSM), and the American Council on Exercise (ACE).

To find out more about Jorge, visit: **JorgeCruise.com.**

We hope you enjoyed this Hay House book. If you'd like to receive our online catalog featuring additional information on Hay House books and products, or if you'd like to find out more about the Hay Foundation, please contact:

Hay House, Inc., P.O. Box 5100, Carlsbad, CA 92018-5100
(760) 431-7695 or **(800) 654-5126**
(760) 431-6948 (fax) or **(800) 650-5115 (fax)**
www.hayhouse.com® • **www.hayfoundation.org**

• • •

Published and distributed in Australia by:
Hay House Australia Pty. Ltd., 18/36 Ralph St., Alexandria NSW 2015
Phone: 612-9669-4299 • *Fax:* 612-9669-4144 • www.hayhouse.com.au

Published and distributed in the United Kingdom by:
Hay House UK, Ltd., 292B Kensal Rd., London W10 5BE • *Phone:* 44-20-8962-1230
Fax: 44-20-8962-1239 • www.hayhouse.co.uk

Published and distributed in the Republic of South Africa by:
Hay House SA (Pty), Ltd., P.O. Box 990, Witkoppen 2068
Phone/Fax: 27-11-467-8904 • www.hayhouse.co.za

Published in India by:
Hay House Publishers India, Muskaan Complex, Plot No. 3, B-2, Vasant Kunj, New Delhi 110 070
Phone: 91-11-4176-1620 • *Fax:* 91-11-4176-1630 • www.hayhouse.co.in

Distributed in Canada by:
Raincoast, 9050 Shaughnessy St., Vancouver, B.C. V6P 6E5
Phone: (604) 323-7100 • *Fax:* (604) 323-2600 • www.raincoast.com

• • •

Take Your Soul on a Vacation

Visit **www.HealYourLife.com**® to regroup, recharge, and reconnect with your own magnificence.
Featuring blogs, mind-body-spirit news, and life-changing wisdom from Louise Hay and friends.

Visit **www.HealYourLife.com** today!

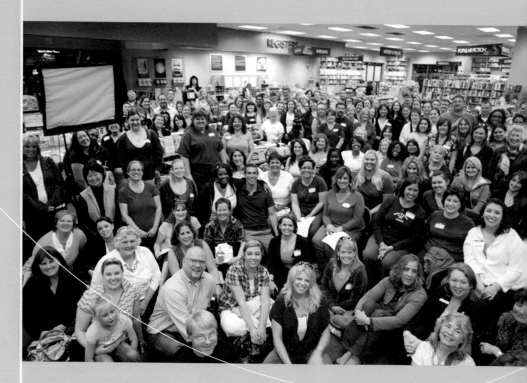